365 Great Cookies and Brownies

Joanne Lamb Hayes
and
Bonnie Tandy Leblang

A John Boswell Associates Book

D0920898

HarperPaperbacks
A Division of HarperCollinsPublishers

If you purchased this book without a cover, you should be aware that this book is stolen property. It was reported as "unsold and destroyed" to the publisher and neither the author nor the publisher has received any payment for this "stripped book."

HarperPaperbacks   *A Division of* HarperCollins*Publishers*
            10 East 53rd Street, New York, N.Y. 10022

Copyright © 1993 by John Boswell Management, Inc. All rights reserved. No part of this book may be used or reproduced in any manner whatsoever without written permission of the publisher, except in the case of brief quotations embodied in critical articles and reviews. For information address HarperCollins*Publishers,* 10 East 53rd Street, New York, N.Y. 10022.

A hardcover edition of this book was published in 1993 by HarperCollins*Publishers.*

Cover design and illustration © 1993 by Rick Rossiter
Text design by Nigel Rollings
Index by Maro Riofrancos

First HarperPaperbacks printing: January 1996

Printed in the United States of America

HarperPaperbacks and colophon are trademarks of HarperCollins*Publishers*

10 9 8 7 6 5 4 3 2 1

Contents

Drop cookies are so fast to make and delicious to sample that we predict many cooking smudges on the pages of this chapter. Try Blueberry Lemon Drops, Molasses Macaroons, Low-Fat Oatmeal Raisin Cookies, and keep on going through Black Walnut Kisses, Lace Cookies, and more.

Rolled cookies are a labor of love that remind family and friends how very special they are. Try Rolled Sugar Cookies or Crisp Ginger Cookies, cutting them with seasonal cookie cutters or into funny shapes for kids. Make cookie sandwiches stuffed with jelly or frosting. On busy evenings, roll out a round of Sugar 'n' Spice Cookies or Oatmeal Shortbread and just score the dough into wedge-shaped cookies.

Shaped cookies, such as Lemon Pretzels, Chocolate Spritz Cookies, Almond Crescents, Sesame Breakfast Rings, Hidden Treasures, and Surprise Shortbread, are fun to make. Invite the children to help, and you will all have a good time.

Icebox or refrigerator cookies were Grandma's quick trick for keeping the cookie jar filled. Make up several recipes at once, refrigerate or freeze the rolls of dough, and then slice and bake them as needed. Try Butterscotch Pennies, Peach Blossoms, Chocolate Coconut Pinwheels, or Ginger Slices and bask in the accolades.

A whole chapter devoted to America's favorite, chocolate chip cookies. From Brickle Chocolate Chip Bars to Chocolate Chunk Butterscotch Cookies, Mint Chocolate Chip Cookies, and many, many more.

Light and dark, fudgy and cakelike, just plain or loaded with extra goodies, here is everything you have always wanted to know about brownies and couldn't wait to sink your teeth into. Take a bite out of Blackout Brownies,

Chocolate Chunk Fudgy Brownies, German Chocolate Brownies, or Chocolate Almond Decadence, just for starters.

In this chapter we examine the age-old question, "Are blondies more fun?" Try Traditional Blondies and a baker's dozen more golden treats, such as Peanut Butter Blondies, Cinnamon Blondies, and Butterscotch Toffee Bars before making your decision.

A whole collection of fruit-filled squares and bars as alluring as the apple that got Eve into trouble. You'll be tempted by Apricot Bars, Linzer Bars, First Date Bars, Oatmeal Date Squares, Apple Walnut Bars, and more.

Pour or pat them into a pan; bake, cut, and enjoy. This chapter is full of all the easy-to-make, cut-up cookies that can't be called brownies. You'll love Cheesecake Squares, Lemon Bites, Chocolate Hazelnut Bars, Peppermint Squares, and Peanut Butter Bars.

Look to this chapter for a taste of the past. Colonial standbys such as Shortenin' Bread and Gingersnaps are joined by nineteenth-century confections, such as Snickerdoodles and Raspberry Tea Cakes, and twentieth-century family fare, such as the Original Toll House Cookies and Oatmeal Raisin Cookies.

Here are the Old World specialties that came to this hemisphere along with the hopes and dreams of three centuries of immigrants: Amaretti, Madeleines, Mexican Anise Cookies, Speculaas, Cream Cheese Rugelach, and Pistachio Biscotti, to name just a few.

Holidays bring to mind special cookie classics. Look here for recipes like Gingerbread Men and Women, Pfeffernüsse, Chocolate Leaf Cookies, Kringles, Robin's Nests, and Candy Canes, to continue a delicious tradition.

Baking Great Cookies and Brownies

Cookies are one of America's favorite desserts. They are portable, packageable, palate-pleasing, and portion controlled. If you want just a little dessert, have a cookie. If you're in the mood for something more, have a handful.

In testing the recipes for this book, we chose to use **butter** unless another shortening is traditional. You can use either sweet or lightly salted butter, but don't use whipped—save that for spreading on your toast. Unless the recipe states otherwise, have the butter softened at room temperature so it is easier to blend in with the other ingredients. Softened butter should be malleable, but not oily.

Lightly grease cookie sheets with either vegetable shortening or vegetable cooking spray. Do not use butter; the salt and moisture might cause cookies to stick.

When a recipe calls for oil, use any light-flavored oil, such as corn, sunflower, canola, light olive, or peanut. Do not substitute oil for butter or other fat in a recipe.

We use unsifted all-purpose **flour**, either bleached or unbleached, for most of our recipes. When measuring flour, we suggest the sweep and level method. Dip the measuring cup into the flour, then level it off using the back of a knife. When a more delicate cookie was desired, we used cake flour. Occasionally for more hearty cookies, we added whole wheat flour or cornmeal to the all-purpose flour.

For all our recipes, we use large **eggs**. It's best to bring eggs to room temperature before using them. If you forget to take them out of the refrigerator, just place them in a bowl of warm water for a few minutes, until they no longer feel cold. It's easiest to separate the yolks from the whites when the eggs are chilled. But for the most volume when whipped, egg whites should be at room temperature before beating. It's also important to use immaculately clean beaters and bowls when working with egg whites. Just a drop of fat can inhibit the egg whites from whipping properly and becoming stiff.

We used many types of **chocolate** for our recipes. Before starting a recipe, check to be sure you have the type of chocolate called for. When a recipe calls for cocoa, use the unsweetened kind; do not use instant cocoa mix. We use semisweet real chocolate chips, chunks, and mini chips for our cookies and brownies. We tested some recipes using semisweet mint chocolate chips, peanut butter chips, and vanilla chips, too.

Unsweetened chocolate, often referred to as baking or bitter chocolate, is basically solidified chocolate liquor. It comes packaged in a box in individually wrapped 1-ounce squares. To substitute cocoa for unsweetened chocolate, use

3 tablespoons unsweetened cocoa powder plus 1 tablespoon butter or shortening for each 1-ounce square of chocolate.

To melt chocolate, place pieces in the top of a double boiler over hot, not bubbling, water. Stir frequently until smooth. Or, microwave chocolate in a microwave-safe bowl, uncovered, on High, for 1 to 2 minutes, or until surface is glossy. Let stand a minute and stir until smooth. When microwaved, chocolate tends to hold its shape until stirred.

In most recipes that call for **coconut** we use flaked coconut, which has been lightly sweetened. To toast coconut, spread it on a sheet pan or piece of foil and bake in a 350°F. oven for about 10 minutes, or until it begins to brown, stirring often.

The most important thing about **nuts** is that they're fresh. The flavor from just a handful of not-so-fresh nuts can ruin your cookies or brownies. To keep our nuts fresh, we always store them in the freezer.

Toasting nuts helps bring out their oils and therefore their flavor. To toast, spread on a sheet pan or piece of foil and bake in a 350°F. oven for 5 to 8 minutes, or until pale golden or aromatic, stirring often.

When our recipes call for **zest,** we're referring to the outer colored rind of a citrus fruit—a lemon, lime, orange, or grapefruit. You can use a zester, a special inexpensive tool designed for that purpose, or a swivel-bladed vegetable peeler. Be sure to remove only the colored part of the rind and not any of the bitter white pith underneath. If you use a vegetable peeler, then use a knife to thinly slice or chop the zest.

We feel that it's very important for the best flavor to use pure **vanilla** and other extracts. They cost a bit more, but in our opinion the results are worth it.

You'll notice that an electric mixer is called for in most of our recipes. We feel it produces a lighter cookie dough and more uniform baking results. (It also saves effort for a tired cook.) However, if you prefer to use a large wooden spoon and mix cookies the old-fashioned way, by all means do so. Just be sure the butter is sufficiently softened and all the ingredients are well incorporated as directed in the recipe.

Your selection of baking pans and cookie sheets will affect the size, shape, brownness, and baking time of your cookies. It is important to use the size pan called for in the recipe so that the cookies will bake in the prescribed time. If you use a larger pan the cookies will be thinner and will bake faster. If you use a smaller pan they will be fatter and take longer to bake. Many of the cookies in this book were tested on insulated cookie sheets. These are sheets made of two layers of aluminum with a cushion of air in the center. Cookies are less likely to burn on the bottoms on these kinds of sheets; however, they bake more slowly and will take the longest baking time given. Shiny, single-layer sheets reflect heat and will bake cookies to an even golden brown in less time than the insulated ones. Dark cookie sheets absorb and hold heat and will bake cookies in the shortest amount of time but with light tops and dark bottoms. To get some of the effect of insulated pans with regular cookie sheets, place one sheet on top of another. This can be very helpful if all you have are thin dark pans.

Another important factor in baking perfectly browned cookies is oven placement. Cookies would be best if baked one tray at a time in the center of the oven. Sometimes this is not possible because you are making lots of cookies and need to get as many as possible in the oven at one time. In this case, it is best to bake on two evenly placed racks: one in the top third of the oven, the other in the bottom third. The cookies on the top rack will get reflected heat from the top of the oven and will brown more quickly on top, while the ones on the bottom rack will get reflected heat from the bottom of the oven and brown quickly on the bottoms. It is important, therefore, to change the position of the trays halfway through the baking time so the cookies will bake evenly. It is also important to leave plenty of room around the trays for the circulation of air in the oven. If circulation is blocked, one portion of a tray will bake more quickly than the rest and will overbake by the time the others are done.

With the exception of a few time-consuming cookies, you can prepare most of our creations in 15 minutes or less. We hope that you will have as much fun making—and eating—our 365 cookies and brownies as we did.

A BAKER'S DOZEN COOKIE-MAKING TIPS

1. Check recipe and make sure you have all ingredients before starting.

2. Measure ingredients accurately, using standard measuring cups and spoons.

3. Use metal or plastic cups (measurement is even with top of cup) for dry ingredients.

4. Use glass cups (with space above largest measure) for liquids.

5. Use an oven thermometer to make sure your oven temperature is correct.

6. When making brownies or bars, always use the pan size called for.

7. Separate eggs carefully; even a little yolk in the whites will prevent them from becoming stiff when beaten.

8. Use an unsalted shortening or vegetable cooking spray

for greasing cookie sheets to prevent sticking.

9. Try to make all the cookies on one sheet uniform in thickness and diameter so they will bake in the same time.

10. When baking dropped and shaped cookies, be sure to leave plenty of room between them. (Many of our recipes call for 2 inches.) Cookies can spread a lot, and you want to keep them separate.

11. Check cookies at the minimum time. If necessary, some may be removed and the rest returned to the oven for longer baking.

12. Always cool cookie sheets between batches; placing cookie dough on hot sheets causes excess spreading and uneven baking.

13. Soft cookies may be packed in a tight container while still a bit warm, but crisp cookies must be completely cool before they are packed, or they will soften.

Mail Order Sources for Ingredients and Equipment

American Spoon Foods
1668 Clarion Ave.
P.O. Box 566
Petoskey, MI 49770-0566
(800) 222-5886

Dried cherries and blueberries

King Arthur Flour Baker's Catalogue
Rural Route 2, Box 56
Norwich, VT 05055
(800) 827-6836

All sorts of baker's supplies. Specialty flours and difficult-to-find baking ingredients, pans, and equipment

Maid of Scandinavia
3244 Raleigh Ave.
Minneapolis, MN 55416
(800) 328-6722

Baking equipment and ingredients. Krumkake irons, rosette irons, cake and cookie decorating supplies

Missouri Dandy Pantry
212 Hammons Drive East
Stockton, MO 65785
(417) 276-5121

Black walnuts

Saco Foods
6120 University Ave.
P.O. Box 616
Madison, WI 53562
(800) 373-SACO (7226)

Dried buttermilk, chocolate chunks, blended cocoa

Walnut Acres
Penns Creek, PA 17862
(800) 433-3998

Unsweetened granola, organic flours, dried fruit, nuts, and seeds

Williams-Sónoma
P.O. Box 7456
San Francisco, CA 94120
(800) 541-2233

Baking pans, housewares, and specialty foods

Wilton Enterprises, Inc.
2240 West 75th St.
Woodbridge, IL 60517
(800) 772-7100 (outside Illinois)

Baking pans, cake decorating equipment, cookie and candy molds

Chapter 1

A Spoonful of Sweetness

Drop cookies are the stir-them-up, pop-them-in-the-oven, and eat-them-right-away kind of cookies. Most likely the first cookies you ever baked were drop cookies and they still hold the record as the type of cookies most often baked in America.

The difference between drop cookies and rolled or refrigerator cookies is in the proportion of flour to moistening ingredients. Because the dough is softer, drop cookies will spread out more than other kinds and should be placed at least 2 inches apart on the cookie sheet.

Drop cookies also tend to be thicker than most other kinds of cookies, so your selection of cookie sheets is more important when baking them. We have included a range of baking times for all the recipes in this book because various factors affect the time it takes to bake cookies to perfection. One of the most important factors is the cookie sheets you bake them on. See page 2 for information on selecting and using cookie sheets.

Most of the recipes in this chapter call for dropping heaping teaspoonfuls of dough onto the cookie sheets. Unless we have specifically called for a measuring teaspoon, we have used a dinnerware teaspoon. "Heaping" means that we have used about twice the amount of dough that would fit in a level teaspoon. If we say "slightly rounded," we have used about 1½ times that in a level measure. Drop cookies are most untemperamental. If you have a little more or a little less dough in each cookie, the only thing that will be affected is the number of cookies. This is why the yield on most of the recipes uses the word "about."

Although we call for mixing doughs with an electric beater, most drop cookie dough is soft enough to be mixed with a fork or a wooden spoon. Even if you have a minimum of cooking equipment, you and your family can enjoy the easy pleasure of home-baked drop cookies warm from the oven.

1   APPLE OATMEAL-RAISIN COOKIES

Prep: 10 minutes   Bake: 15 to 18 minutes   Makes: about 40

Cinnamon and apples turn these traditional oatmeal cookies into a fall delight. Granny Smiths are a good choice to use here.

2 cups firmly packed dark brown sugar	1 teaspoon grated nutmeg
2 sticks (8 ounces) butter, softened	1 teaspoon cinnamon
	½ teaspoon baking soda
2 eggs	¼ teaspoon salt
1 teaspoon vanilla extract	1½ cups finely diced, peeled tart cooking apples
2¼ cups flour	1 cup raisins
2 cups rolled oats	1 cup chopped walnuts
1 teaspoon baking powder	

1. Preheat oven to 375°F. In a large bowl, beat brown sugar and butter with an electric mixer on medium speed until light and fluffy. Beat in eggs and vanilla until well blended.

2. Add flour mixed with oatmeal, baking powder, nutmeg, cinnamon, baking soda, and salt to butter-sugar mixture and beat until well blended. Stir in apples, raisins, and walnuts. Drop by teaspoonfuls onto greased cookie sheets.

3. Bake 15 to 18 minutes, just until edges begin to brown. Let cookies cool 2 minutes on sheets, then remove to a rack and let cool completely.

---

2   BLACK WALNUT KISSES

Prep: 10 minutes   Bake: 10 minutes   Stand: 2 hours
Makes: about 24

Sometimes a kiss is not just a kiss. When you bite through the crisp exterior of these meringue drops, you find a chewy walnut center.

2 egg whites, at room temperature	⅔ cup sugar
	½ cup chopped black walnuts
½ teaspoon cream of tartar	½ teaspoon vanilla extract
¼ teaspoon salt	

1. Preheat oven to 275°F. In a small bowl, beat egg whites, cream of tartar, and salt with an electric mixer on high speed until frothy. Very slowly beat in sugar, a little at a time, until all has been incorporated and whites are very stiff. Fold in black walnuts and vanilla.

2. Drop by heaping teaspoonfuls 2 inches apart onto generously greased cookie sheets. Bake 10 minutes. Turn off oven and let cookies stand in closed oven for 2 hours. Remove cookies from sheets and store in a tightly covered container.

3   BANANA GRANOLA COOKIES
Prep: 5 minutes   Bake: 12 to 15 minutes   Makes: about 40

1 stick (4 ounces) butter, softened
¼ cup solid vegetable shortening
1 cup firmly packed dark brown sugar
½ cup mashed banana (about 1 medium)
1 egg
1 teaspoon vanilla extract

½ teaspoon banana extract (optional)
2 cups granola
1½ cups flour
½ teaspoon salt
½ teaspoon baking powder
½ teaspoon cinnamon
½ teaspoon grated nutmeg
½ cup semisweet mini chocolate chips

1. Preheat oven to 400°F. In a medium bowl, beat butter, shortening, and brown sugar with an electric mixer on medium speed until creamy. Beat in banana, egg, vanilla, and banana extract until well blended.

2. Add granola, flour, salt, baking powder, cinnamon, and nutmeg and mix until blended. Stir in chocolate chips.

3. Drop teaspoonfuls of dough 2 inches apart onto lightly greased cookie sheets. Bake 12 to 15 minutes, just until lightly brown. Remove to a rack to cool completely.

4   BLUEBERRY LEMON DROPS
Prep: 10 minutes   Bake: 12 to 15 minutes   Makes: about 36

Dried blueberries are available in specialty food shops or they can be ordered through the mail (see page 4).

1 stick (4 ounces) butter, softened
1 cup sugar
1 egg
½ teaspoon lemon extract
2 teaspoons grated lemon zest

2 cups flour
1 teaspoon baking powder
¼ teaspoon salt
¼ cup milk
⅔ cup dried blueberries (about 3 ounces)

1. Preheat oven to 350°F. In a large bowl, beat butter and sugar with an electric mixer on medium speed until creamy. Add egg, lemon extract, and lemon zest and beat until well blended.

2. Add flour, baking powder, and salt to sugar mixture alternately with milk until well blended. Stir in blueberries. Drop by teaspoonfuls 2 inches apart onto greased cookie sheets.

3. Bake 12 to 15 minutes. Let cookies cool on sheets 2 minutes, then remove to a rack and let cool completely.

5   BONANZA BLASTS
Prep: 10 minutes   Bake: 12 to 14 minutes   Makes: about 30

These chewy cookies are enriched with lots of extras: coconut, chocolate, nuts, and cereal.

1 cup firmly packed dark brown sugar	½ teaspoon salt
2 sticks (8 ounces) butter, softened	1 cup rolled oats
2 eggs	½ cup crushed cereal (cornflakes or bran flakes)
1 teaspoon vanilla extract	1 cup semisweet mini chocolate chips (6 ounces)
2 cups flour	½ cup finely chopped pecans
1 teaspoon baking powder	½ cup flaked coconut

1. Preheat oven to 350°F. In a medium bowl, beat brown sugar and butter with an electric mixer on medium speed until fluffy. Beat in eggs and vanilla until well blended.

2. Add flour, baking powder, and salt to the sugar mixture until well blended. Stir in oatmeal, cereal, chocolate chips, pecans, and coconut. Drop by teaspoonfuls onto greased cookie sheets.

3. Bake 12 to 14 minutes, or until edges begin to brown. Let cookies cool 2 minutes on sheets, then remove to a rack and let cool completely.

---

6   BUTTER PECAN COOKIES
Prep: 10 minutes   Bake: 12 to 15 minutes   Makes: about 24

The aroma of butter, brown sugar, and pecans baking together entices everyone to the kitchen before these cookies are out of the oven. You might want to double this recipe.

1 stick (4 ounces) butter, softened	1 cup flour
⅓ cup firmly packed brown sugar	¼ teaspoon salt
1 egg yolk	½ teaspoon vanilla extract
	24 pecan halves, or as needed

1. Preheat oven to 350°F. In a large bowl, beat butter and brown sugar with an electric mixer on medium speed until well blended. Beat in egg yolk until light and fluffy.

2. On low speed, beat in flour, salt, and vanilla until dough is smooth, scraping side of bowl frequently with a rubber spatula.

3. Drop dough by slightly rounded teaspoonfuls 2 inches apart onto lightly greased cookie sheets. Press a pecan half into center of each. Bake 12 to 15 minutes, or until edges are golden brown. Let cookies cool 2 minutes on sheets, then remove to racks and let cool completely. Store in a tightly covered container.

7   CARROT COOKIES

Prep: 15 minutes   Bake: 12 to 15 minutes   Makes: about 30

The sweetness of carrots and raisins makes these soft cookies the perfect after-school partners for a large frosty glass of milk.

½ cup firmly packed brown
  sugar
1 stick (4 ounces) butter,
  softened
1 egg
1 teaspoon grated orange zest

1 cup flour
1 teaspoon baking powder
¼ teaspoon salt
1 cup shredded raw carrots
  (about 3)
¼ cup raisins

1. Preheat oven to 350°F. In a large bowl, beat brown sugar and butter with an electric mixer on medium speed until well blended. Beat in egg and orange zest until light and fluffy.

2. Beat in flour mixed with baking powder and salt until dough is smooth, scraping sides of bowl frequently with a rubber scraper. Fold in carrots and raisins.

3. Drop dough by heaping teaspoonfuls 2 inches apart onto lightly greased cookie sheets. Bake 12 to 15 minutes, or until golden brown. Let cookies cool 2 minutes on sheets, then remove to racks and let cool completely. Store in a tightly covered container in refrigerator.

8   CASHEW DROPS

Prep: 10 minutes   Bake: 10 to 12 minutes   Makes: about 44

Raw cashews can be found in health food stores, and they can be ordered by mail from Walnut Acres (see page 4).

1 stick (4 ounces) butter,
  softened
⅔ cup firmly packed brown
  sugar
1 egg
1 teaspoon vanilla extract

1½ cups flour
½ teaspoon baking powder
½ teaspoon baking soda
¼ teaspoon salt
1½ cups broken raw cashew
  nuts

1. Preheat oven to 350°F. In a large bowl, beat butter and brown sugar with an electric mixer on medium speed until well blended. Beat in egg and vanilla until light and fluffy.

2. Beat in flour mixed with baking powder, soda, and salt until dough is smooth, scraping side of bowl frequently with a rubber spatula. Fold in cashews. Drop by heaping teaspoonfuls 2 inches apart onto lightly greased cookie sheets.

3. Bake 10 to 12 minutes, or until golden brown. Let cookies cool 2 minutes on sheets, then remove to racks and let cool completely. Store in a tightly covered container.

9   BRANDY SNAPS
Prep: 10 minutes   Bake: 6 to 8 minutes   Makes: about 38

These crisp lacy cookies are delicately flavored with brandy.

4 tablespoons butter, softened	½ cup cake flour
¼ cup sugar	⅛ teaspoon salt
¼ cup brandy	

1. Preheat oven to 350°F. In a medium bowl, beat butter and sugar with an electric mixer on medium speed until well blended. Beat in brandy; then beat in flour and salt until a soft dough forms, scraping down sides of bowl frequently with a rubber spatula.

2. Drop by slightly rounded measuring teaspoonfuls 3 inches apart on well-greased cookie sheets. Bake 6 to 8 minutes, or until golden brown at edges.

3. Let cookies cool 1 minute on sheets, then remove to racks and let cool completely. Store in a tightly covered container.

10   CHOCOLATE ALMOND KISS COOKIES
Prep: 10 minutes   Bake: 10 to 12 minutes   Makes: about 54

1 stick (4 ounces) butter, softened	1 teaspoon baking powder
½ cup sugar	¼ teaspoon salt
2 eggs	½ cup sliced natural almonds
1 teaspoon almond extract	1 (9-ounce) package milk chocolate kisses with almonds
2 cups flour	

1. Preheat oven to 350°F. In a large bowl, beat butter and sugar with an electric mixer on medium speed until light and fluffy. Beat in eggs and almond extract until well blended.

2. Beat in flour mixed with baking powder and salt until dough is smooth, scraping down side of bowl frequently with a rubber spatula. Fold in sliced almonds.

3. Drop by heaping measuring teaspoonfuls 2 inches apart onto lightly greased cookie sheets. Press dough to flatten slightly.

4. Bake 8 minutes. Meanwhile, remove foil wrappers from kisses. Remove cookies from oven, leaving oven on. Carefully press a kiss pointed side up into center of each cookie. Return to oven and bake 2 to 4 minutes longer, or until golden brown. Let cookies cool 2 minutes on sheets, then remove to racks and let cool completely. Store in a tightly covered container.

11   CHOCOLATE BANANA COOKIES
Prep: 10 minutes   Bake: 8 to 10 minutes   Makes: about 30

These small, banana-flavored cookies are more like moist mini cakes than cookies.

1 stick (4 ounces) unsalted
   butter, softened
¾ cup firmly packed dark
   brown sugar
1 egg
1 teaspoon vanilla extract
¾ cup mashed bananas (about
   2 medium)

1 (4-ounce) bar sweet
   chocolate, melted
1¾ cups flour
1 teaspoon baking powder
¼ teaspoon salt

1. Preheat oven to 400°F. In a medium bowl, beat butter and brown sugar with an electric mixer on medium speed until creamy. Beat in egg and vanilla until well blended. Stir in bananas and chocolate.

2. Mix flour, baking powder, and salt. Add to sugar mixture and stir until blended.

3. Drop teaspoonfuls of dough 2 inches apart onto greased cookie sheets. Bake 8 to 10 minutes, just until edges of cookies start to brown. Let cookies cool on sheets 2 minutes, then remove to a rack and let cool completely.

12   CHOCOLATE DROPS
Prep: 10 minutes   Bake: 8 to 10 minutes   Makes: about 36

¾ cup sugar
¼ cup vegetable oil
2 (1-ounce) squares
   unsweetened chocolate,
   melted
1 egg

1 teaspoon vanilla extract
1 cup flour
1 teaspoon baking powder
¼ teaspoon salt
½ cup chopped walnuts

1. Preheat oven to 350°F. In a large bowl, beat sugar, oil, and chocolate with an electric mixer on medium speed until well blended. Beat in egg and vanilla until light and fluffy.

2. Beat in flour, baking powder, and salt until dough is smooth, scraping down side of bowl frequently with a rubber spatula. Fold in walnuts.

3. Drop dough by heaping teaspoonfuls 2 inches apart onto lightly greased cookie sheets. Bake 8 to 10 minutes, or until firm in center. Let cookies cool 2 minutes on sheets, then remove to racks to cool completely. Store in a tightly covered container.

13   CHOCOLATE SNAPS
Prep: 10 minutes   Bake: 6 to 8 minutes   Makes: about 40

4 tablespoons butter, softened	**½ cup flour**
⅓ cup sugar	**¼ cup unsweetened cocoa**
1 egg	**powder**
1 teaspoon vanilla extract	**¼ teaspoon salt**

1. Preheat oven to 350°F. In a large bowl, beat butter and sugar with an electric mixer on medium speed until well blended. Beat in egg and vanilla until light and fluffy.

2. Beat in flour, cocoa powder, and salt until dough is smooth, scraping down side of bowl frequently with a rubber spatula.

3. Drop by slightly rounded measuring teaspoonfuls 3 inches apart onto well-greased cookie sheets. Flatten slightly with floured back of a spoon.

4. Bake 6 to 8 minutes, or until cookies are firm and tops look dry. Let snaps cool 1 minute on sheets, then remove to racks and let cool completely. Store in a tightly covered container.

---

14   COCOA SPICE DROPS
Prep: 10 minutes   Bake: 12 to 15 minutes   Makes: about 36

Sweet spices enhance the cocoa flavor of these crisp cookies.

¾ cup firmly packed brown	**½ teaspoon baking soda**
sugar	**½ teaspoon cinnamon**
1 stick (4 ounces) butter,	**¼ teaspoon ground cloves**
softened	**¼ teaspoon salt**
1 egg	**½ cup chopped walnuts**
1¼ cups flour	**1 (1-ounce) square semisweet**
¼ cup unsweetened cocoa	**chocolate, melted**
powder	

1. Preheat oven to 350°F. In a large bowl, beat brown sugar and butter with an electric mixer on medium speed until well blended. Beat in egg until light and fluffy.

2. Mix flour with cocoa powder, baking soda, cinnamon, cloves, and salt. Beat into butter mixture until dough is smooth, scraping down side of bowl frequently with a rubber spatula. Fold in walnuts.

3. Drop dough by heaping teaspoonfuls 2 inches apart onto lightly greased cookie sheets. Bake 12 to 15 minutes, or until golden brown. Let cookies cool 2 minutes on sheets, then remove to racks. Drizzle melted chocolate over tops of cookies and set aside to cool completely. Store in a tightly covered container.

15   AUNT MIL'S GOOD COOKIES
Prep: 10 minutes   Bake: 9 to 10 minutes   Makes: about 44

Joanne got this recipe from her aunt, Mildred Myers. Perhaps there is another name for them, but everyone in the family has always called them Aunt Mil's Good Cookies.

1 stick (4 ounces) butter, softened	½ teaspoon baking powder
½ cup granulated sugar	¼ teaspoon baking soda
½ cup firmly packed brown sugar	¼ teaspoon salt
	1 cup crisp rice cereal
1 egg	½ cup rolled oats
1 teaspoon vanilla extract	½ cup flaked coconut
¾ cup flour	¼ cup chopped pecans

1. Preheat oven to 350°F. In a large bowl, beat butter, granulated sugar, and brown sugar with an electric mixer on medium speed until well blended. Beat in egg and vanilla until light and fluffy.

2. Beat in flour mixed with baking powder, soda, and salt until dough is smooth, scraping down side of bowl frequently with a rubber spatula. Fold in rice cereal, oatmeal, coconut, and pecans. Drop by heaping teaspoonfuls 2 inches apart onto lightly greased cookie sheets.

3. Bake 9 to 10 minutes, or until golden brown. Let cookies cool 2 minutes on sheets, then remove to racks and let cool completely. Store in a tightly covered container.

16   COCOA LACE COOKIES
Prep: 10 minutes   Bake: 5 to 6 minutes   Makes: about 36

1 stick (4 ounces) butter, softened	⅔ cup flour
½ cup sugar	¼ cup unsweetened cocoa powder
⅓ cup light corn syrup	¼ teaspoon salt
1 teaspoon vanilla extract	1 cup rolled oats

1. Preheat oven to 350°F. In a medium bowl, beat butter, sugar, corn syrup, and vanilla with an electric mixer on medium speed until well blended. Beat in flour, cocoa powder, and salt until batter is smooth. Fold in oatmeal.

2. Drop by level teaspoonfuls 3 inches apart onto generously greased cookie sheets. Flatten slightly with back of spoon. Bake 5 to 6 minutes, or until golden brown around edges. Let cookies cool 1 minute on sheets, then remove to racks and let cool completely. Store in a tightly covered container.

17   FLORENTINES
Prep: 10 minutes   Bake: 10 to 12 minutes   Makes: about 40

1   stick (4 ounces) butter,
    softened
¼   cup sugar
1   teaspoon vanilla extract
¼   cup plus 2 tablespoons flour
¼   cup milk

½   cup sliced blanched
    almonds
¼   cup finely chopped candied
    orange peel
4   (1-ounce) squares semisweet
    or bittersweet chocolate,
    melted

1. Preheat oven to 350°F. In a medium bowl, beat butter, sugar, and vanilla with an electric mixer on medium speed until well blended. Beat in flour and milk until a soft dough forms. Fold in almonds and orange peel.

2. Drop by slightly rounded measuring teaspoonfuls 3 inches apart onto generously greased cookie sheets. Flatten slightly with floured back of a spoon to make 2-inch rounds.

3. Bake 10 to 12 minutes, or until golden brown around edges. Let cookies cool 1 minute on sheets, then remove to racks and let cool completely.

4. Turn cooled cookies upside down and spread a thin layer of melted chocolate over bottoms. Let cool until chocolate is firm. Store in a tightly covered container.

---

18   GINGER WAFERS
Prep: 10 minutes   Bake: 6 to 8 minutes   Makes: about 60

Fresh ginger gives an exotic nip to these paper-thin cookies.

4   tablespoons butter, softened
¾   cup powdered sugar
⅓   cup honey
¾   cup flour

¼   teaspoon salt
1   egg
1   tablespoon finely shredded
    fresh ginger

1. Preheat oven to 350°F. In a medium bowl, beat butter and powdered sugar with an electric mixer on medium speed until well blended. Beat in honey, flour, salt, and egg until a smooth batter forms. Fold in ginger.

2. Drop by slightly rounded measuring teaspoonfuls 2 inches apart onto lightly greased cookie sheets.

3. Bake 6 to 8 minutes, or until edges begin to brown. Let wafers cool 2 minutes on sheets, then remove to racks and let cool completely. Store in a tightly covered container.

19   FRUIT, GRAIN, AND COCONUT COOKIES
Prep: 10 minutes   Bake: 12 to 15 minutes   Makes: about 36

Between the raisins and wheat cereal, these soft cookies are iron enriched.

1 cup whole wheat flour
½ cup all-purpose flour
½ cup farina (Cream of Wheat cereal)
1½ teaspoons baking powder
½ teaspoon grated nutmeg
¼ teaspoon salt

1½ sticks (6 ounces) butter, softened
¾ cup sugar
1 egg, at room temperature
1 teaspoon vanilla extract
½ cup flaked coconut
½ cup golden raisins

1. Preheat oven to 350°F. In a small bowl, combine whole wheat flour, all-purpose flour, farina, baking powder, nutmeg, and salt.

2. In a medium bowl, beat butter and sugar with an electric mixer on medium speed until light and fluffy. Beat in egg and vanilla.

3. Add flour mixture to butter-sugar mixture and beat until blended. Stir in coconut and raisins. Drop dough by teaspoonfuls 2 inches apart onto greased cookie sheets. Bake 12 to 15 minutes, until cookies are set and edges begin to brown. Let cookies cool on sheets 2 minutes, then remove to a rack and let cool completely.

20   HONEY DROPS
Prep: 10 minutes   Bake: 12 to 15 minutes   Makes: about 30

Be careful to mix these just until the flour has been moistened. Overmixing can make them tough.

½ cup honey
1 stick (4 ounces) butter, softened
2 teaspoons grated orange zest

1¾ cups flour
2 teaspoons baking powder
¼ teaspoon salt
1 cup finely chopped walnuts

1. Preheat oven to 350°F. In a large bowl, beat honey, butter, and orange zest with an electric mixer on medium speed until light and fluffy.

2. Stir in flour mixed with baking powder and salt until just blended, scraping down side of bowl frequently with a rubber spatula. Fold in walnuts.

3. Drop dough by heaping teaspoonfuls 2 inches apart onto lightly greased cookie sheets. Press slightly with floured back of teaspoon to flatten.

4. Bake 12 to 15 minutes, or until golden brown. Let cookies cool 2 minutes on sheets, then remove to a rack and let cool completely. Store in a tightly covered container.

21   COCONUT WHEAT COOKIES
Prep: 10 minutes   Bake: 12 to 15 minutes   Makes: about 36

This recipe dates back to the days when adding cereal was an inexpensive way to extend cookie dough.

1½ sticks (6 ounces) butter, softened	1½ cups flour
¾ cup granulated sugar	½ teaspoon baking powder
¾ cup firmly packed brown sugar	¼ teaspoon baking soda
2 eggs	¼ teaspoon salt
½ teaspoon vanilla extract	2 cups flaked wheat cereal, such as Wheaties
	¾ cup flaked coconut

1. Preheat oven to 350°F. In a large bowl, beat butter, granulated sugar, and brown sugar with an electric mixer on medium speed until well blended. Beat in eggs and vanilla until light and fluffy.

2. Beat in flour, baking powder, soda, and salt until dough is smooth, scraping down side of bowl frequently with a rubber spatula. Fold in wheat cereal and coconut. Drop by heaping teaspoonfuls 2 inches apart onto lightly greased cookie sheets.

3. Bake 12 to 15 minutes, or until golden brown. Let cookies cool 2 minutes on sheets, then remove to racks and let cool completely. Store in a tightly covered container.

22   LACE COOKIES
Prep: 10 minutes   Bake: 5 to 6 minutes   Makes: about 40

The trick to successful lace cookies is allowing them to cool just enough to be manageable, but not so much that they are stiff and crack when removed from pans or rolled.

1 stick (4 ounces) butter	1 cup finely chopped hazelnuts or natural almonds
½ cup firmly packed brown sugar	
⅓ cup light corn syrup	1 teaspoon vanilla extract
1 cup flour	¼ teaspoon salt

1. Preheat oven to 375°F. In a medium saucepan, combine butter, brown sugar, and corn syrup. Bring to a boil over medium heat, stirring constantly. Remove from heat and stir in flour, hazelnuts, vanilla, and salt.

2. Drop by teaspoonfuls 3 inches apart onto generously greased cookie sheets. Bake 5 to 6 minutes, or until golden brown. Let cookies cool 1 minute on sheets, then remove to racks and let cool completely, or roll around the handle of a wooden spoon and slide off onto racks to cool completely. Store in a tightly covered container.

23   KITCHEN SINK COOKIES
Prep: 10 minutes   Bake: 12 to 15 minutes   Makes: about 40

As you can tell from the name, these cookies have an incredible amount of goodies mixed into them.

1 stick (4 ounces) butter, softened
¾ cup sugar
2 eggs
1 teaspoon vanilla extract
2 tablespoons milk
1 cup flour
1 cup rolled oats
1 teaspoon baking powder
1 teaspoon cinnamon
½ teaspoon salt
1 cup chopped walnuts
1 cup flaked coconut
1 cup raisins
1 cup semisweet chocolate chips (6 ounces)
1 cup dried cranberries
½ cup finely chopped pitted dates

1. Preheat oven to 350°F. In a medium bowl, beat butter and sugar with an electric mixer on medium speed until light and fluffy. Beat in eggs, vanilla, and milk.

2. Mix flour and oatmeal with baking powder, cinnamon, and salt. Add to sugar mixture and beat until blended. Stir in walnuts, coconut, raisins, chocolate chips, cranberries, and dates.

3. Drop teaspoonfuls of dough 2 inches apart onto ungreased cookie sheets. Bake 12 to 15 minutes, just until edges begin to brown. Let cookies cool 2 minutes on sheets, then remove to a rack and let cool completely.

24   LOW-FAT OATMEAL RAISIN COOKIES
Prep: 10 minutes   Bake: 10 to 12 minutes   Makes: about 42

⅔ cup pitted prunes
¾ cup flour
½ cup firmly packed brown sugar
1 teaspoon cinnamon
½ teaspoon baking soda
¼ teaspoon salt
2 egg whites
¼ cup honey
1¼ cups rolled oats
½ cup raisins

1. Preheat oven to 350°F. In a food processor or blender, puree prunes until smooth.

2. In a large bowl, stir together flour, brown sugar, cinnamon, baking soda, and salt. Add prune puree, egg whites, and honey. Beat with an electric mixer on medium speed until well blended, scraping down side of bowl frequently with a rubber spatula. Fold in oatmeal and raisins.

3. Drop dough by heaping teaspoonfuls 2 inches apart onto lightly greased cookie sheets. Bake 10 to 12 minutes, or until golden brown. Let cookies cool 2 minutes on sheets, then remove to racks and let cool completely. Store in a tightly covered container.

25   LOW-FAT MOLASSES RAISIN COOKIES
Prep: 10 minutes   Bake: 10 to 12 minutes   Makes: about 36

The substitution of prune puree for shortening makes these sweet, chewy cookies very low in fat.

⅔ cup pitted prunes (4 ounces)
2 cups flour
½ cup firmly packed brown sugar
1½ teaspoons ground ginger
1 teaspoon cinnamon
1 teaspoon baking soda

¼ teaspoon ground cloves
¼ teaspoon salt
2 egg whites
⅓ cup nonfat plain yogurt
⅓ cup light molasses
½ cup raisins

1. Preheat oven to 350°F. In a food processor, puree prunes until smooth.

2. In a large bowl, stir together flour, brown sugar, ginger, cinnamon, baking soda, cloves, and salt. Add prune puree, egg whites, yogurt, and molasses. Beat with an electric mixer on medium speed until well blended, scraping down side of bowl frequently with a rubber spatula. Fold in raisins. Drop dough by heaping teaspoonfuls 2 inches apart onto lightly greased cookie sheets.

3. Bake 10 to 12 minutes, or until golden brown. Let cookies cool 2 minutes on sheets, then remove to racks and let cool completely. Store in a tightly covered container.

26   OATMEAL GEMS
Prep: 10 minutes   Bake: 15 to 20 minutes   Makes: about 36

1½ cups firmly packed dark brown sugar
1½ sticks (6 ounces) butter, softened
1 egg
1 (8-ounce) can crushed pineapple in juice
1 teaspoon vanilla extract

1 cup flour
½ teaspoon baking powder
½ teaspoon salt
½ teaspoon cinnamon
¼ teaspoon baking soda
¼ teaspoon grated nutmeg
3 cups rolled oats
1 cup raisins

1. Preheat oven to 350°F. In a large bowl, beat brown sugar and butter with an electric mixer on medium speed until light and fluffy. Beat in egg, pineapple with its juice, and vanilla until well blended.

2. Stir in flour mixed with baking powder, salt, cinnamon, baking soda, and nutmeg. Add oatmeal and beat until well blended. Stir in raisins.

3. Drop dough by teaspoonfuls onto greased cookie sheets. Bake 15 to 20 minutes, until golden. Let cookies cool on sheets 2 minutes, then remove to a rack and let cool completely.

27 MOLASSES MACAROONS
Prep: 10 minutes   Bake: 10 to 12 minutes   Makes: about 44

These are a delicious marriage of chewy coconut macaroons and molasses gingersnaps.

1 cup sugar	2 cups flour
1 stick (4 ounces) plus 2 tablespoons butter, softened	1 teaspoon baking soda
	1 teaspoon cinnamon
	1 teaspoon ground ginger
¼ cup light molasses	¼ teaspoon ground cloves
1 egg	½ cup flaked coconut

1. Preheat oven to 350°F. Place ¼ cup sugar in a shallow dish. In a large bowl, beat butter and remaining ¾ cup sugar with an electric mixer on medium speed until well blended. Beat in molasses and egg until light and fluffy.

2. Beat in flour mixed with baking soda, cinnamon, ginger, and cloves until dough is smooth, scraping down side of bowl frequently with a rubber spatula. Fold in coconut.

3. Drop dough by heaping teaspoonfuls into dish of sugar and toss gently to coat. Place 2 inches apart onto lightly greased cookie sheets.

4. Bake 10 to 12 minutes, or until golden brown. Let cookies cool 2 minutes on sheets, then remove to racks and let cool completely. Store in a tightly covered container.

28 PECAN BUTTER COOKIES
Prep: 10 minutes   Chill: 1 hour   Bake: 6 to 8 minutes
Makes: about 30

2 sticks (8 ounces) unsalted butter, softened	1 teaspoon vanilla extract
	1 teaspoon baking soda
½ cup firmly packed dark brown sugar	½ teaspoon salt
	1¼ cups flour
¼ cup granulated sugar	1¼ cups coarsely chopped pecans
1 egg	

1. In a medium bowl, with an electric mixer on medium speed, beat butter, brown sugar, and granulated sugar until creamy. Beat in egg, vanilla, baking soda, and salt until well blended.

2. Add flour to butter-sugar mixture and beat until blended. Stir in the chopped nuts. Cover and refrigerate dough at least 1 hour, until chilled.

3. Preheat oven to 400°F. Drop heaping teaspoons of dough 2 inches apart onto greased cookie sheets. Bake 6 to 8 minutes, just until edges start to brown. Let stand 2 minutes on cookie sheets before removing to a rack to cool completely.

29   OATMEAL DATE DROPS
Prep: 10 minutes   Bake: 15 to 18 minutes   Makes: about 48

These cookies stay moist during storage and ship well.

½ cup firmly packed brown sugar
1 stick (4 ounces) butter, softened
½ cup buttermilk
¼ cup honey
1 egg
1 teaspoon vanilla extract
½ teaspoon almond extract
1 cup flour
½ teaspoon baking soda
¼ teaspoon salt
3 cups rolled oats
1 cup coarsely chopped dates
½ cup slivered almonds

1. Preheat oven to 350°F. In a large bowl, beat brown sugar and butter with an electric mixer on medium speed until light and fluffy. Beat in buttermilk, honey, egg, vanilla, and almond extract until well blended.

2. Mix together flour, baking soda, and salt and beat in until dough is smooth, scraping down side of bowl frequently with a rubber spatula. Stir in oats, dates, and almonds.

3. Drop dough by heaping teaspoonfuls 2 inches apart onto lightly greased cookie sheets. Bake 15 to 18 minutes, or until golden brown. Let cookies cool 2 minutes on sheets, then remove to racks and let cool completely. Store in a tightly covered container.

30   PIGNOLI COOKIES
Prep: 10 minutes   Bake: 20 to 25 minutes   Makes: about 60

These delicious, buttery cookies are a perfect wrapping for those expensive nuts.

1 cup pine nuts (pignoli)
2 sticks (8 ounces) butter, softened
1 cup sugar
1 egg, at room temperature
2 teaspoons vanilla extract
1 teaspoon lemon juice
2 cups flour

1. Preheat oven to 350°F. Spread out pine nuts on a baking sheet. Bake 5 to 7 minutes, shaking pan once or twice, until nuts are lightly browned and fragrant.

2. In a medium bowl, beat butter and sugar with an electric mixer on medium speed until light and fluffy. Beat in egg, vanilla, and lemon juice.

3. Add flour to butter-sugar mixture and beat until blended. Stir in pignoli. Cover and refrigerate at least 1 hour, until firm.

4. Preheat oven to 300°F. Drop batter by teaspoonfuls onto greased cookie sheets. Bake 20 to 25 minutes, or until edges just begin to turn pale golden. Remove to a rack and let cool completely.

31 MAPLE WALNUT COOKIES
Prep: 10 minutes   Bake: 12 to 15 minutes   Makes: about 48

1 stick (4 ounces) butter, softened	¾ cup flour
½ cup firmly packed dark brown sugar	½ cup rolled oats
2 tablespoons maple syrup	¼ teaspoon salt
	½ cup finely chopped walnuts

1. Preheat oven to 350°F. In a medium bowl, beat butter, brown sugar, and maple syrup with an electric mixer on medium speed until light and fluffy.

2. Add flour, oatmeal, and salt to sugar mixture and mix until blended. Stir in walnuts. Drop by teaspoonfuls 2 inches apart onto greased cookie sheets.

3. Bake 12 to 15 minutes, until set. Let cookies cool on sheets 2 minutes, then remove to a rack and let cool completely.

32 PUMPKIN WALNUT COOKIES
Prep: 15 minutes   Bake: 12 to 15 minutes   Makes: about 48

1 stick (4 ounces) butter, softened	1 teaspoon cinnamon
1 cup firmly packed dark brown sugar	½ teaspoon grated nutmeg
¼ cup dark corn syrup	¼ teaspoon ground allspice
1 egg	1 teaspoon baking powder
1 teaspoon vanilla extract	¼ teaspoon salt
1 cup canned pumpkin puree	1 cup currants
2 cups flour	1 cup chopped walnuts
	1 cup powdered sugar
	2 tablespoons orange juice

1. Preheat oven to 350°F. In a medium bowl, beat butter and brown sugar with an electric mixer on medium speed until creamy. Beat in corn syrup, egg, and vanilla, then blend in pumpkin.

2. Mix together flour, cinnamon, nutmeg, allspice, baking powder, and salt. Add to pumpkin mixture and beat until well blended. Stir in currants and ¾ cup walnuts.

3. Drop by heaping teaspoonfuls 1 inch apart onto greased cookie sheets. Bake 12 to 15 minutes, until lightly browned around edges. Let cookies cool on sheets 2 minutes, then remove to a rack and let cool completely.

4. In a small bowl, stir together powdered sugar and orange juice until smooth. Spread glaze over cooled cookies, then sprinkle remaining ¼ cup walnuts on top.

33   PINEAPPLE JEWELS
Prep: 10 minutes   Bake: 12 to 15 minutes   Makes: about 48

1 cup firmly packed dark
   brown sugar
½ cup solid vegetable
   shortening
1 egg
1 teaspoon vanilla extract
1 (8-ounce) can crushed
   pineapple in juice, well
   drained, 2 tablespoons
   juice reserved

2 cups cake flour
2 teaspoons baking powder
½ teaspoon baking soda
¼ teaspoon salt
½ cup flaked coconut
1 cup powdered sugar

1. Preheat oven to 350°F. In a large bowl, beat brown sugar and shortening with an electric mixer on medium speed until light and fluffy. Beat in egg, vanilla, and drained pineapple until well blended.

2. Add cake flour mixed with baking powder, baking soda, and salt and beat until blended. Stir in coconut.

3. Drop by teaspoonfuls onto greased cookie sheets. Bake 12 to 15 minutes. Let cookies cool on sheets 2 minutes, then remove to a rack and let cool completely.

4. In a small bowl, stir together powdered sugar and pineapple juice until blended and smooth. Spread glaze over cooled cookies. Let cool before serving.

---

34   RAISIN-ALMOND WHEAT DROPS
Prep: 10 minutes   Bake: 15 to 20 minutes   Makes: about 36

1½ cups flour
½ cup toasted wheat cereal,
   such as Wheatena
1 teaspoon cinnamon
1½ teaspoons baking powder
¼ teaspoon salt
1½ sticks (6 ounces) butter,
   softened

¾ cup firmly packed dark
   brown sugar
1 egg, at room temperature
1 teaspoon vanilla extract
½ cup toasted slivered
   almonds
½ cup raisins

1. Preheat oven to 350°F. In a small bowl, combine flour, cereal, cinnamon, baking powder, and salt.

2. In a medium bowl, beat butter and brown sugar with an electric mixer on medium speed until light and fluffy. Beat in egg and vanilla.

3. Add flour mixture to butter-sugar mixture and beat until blended. Stir in almonds and raisins. Drop dough by teaspoonfuls 2 inches apart onto greased cookie sheets. Bake 15 to 20 minutes, or until cookies are set and edges begin to brown. Let cookies cool on sheets 2 minutes, then remove to a rack and let cool completely.

35 PIÑA COLADA OATMEAL COOKIES
Prep: 10 minutes   Bake: 15 to 20 minutes   Makes: about 48

Flavored with pineapple, coconut, and rum, these cookies are reminiscent of the rum and pineapple drink, a piña colada.

1½ cups firmly packed dark
    brown sugar
1½ sticks (6 ounces) butter,
    softened
1 egg
1 (8-ounce) can crushed
    pineapple in juice

1 teaspoon rum extract
2 cups flour
½ teaspoon baking powder
¼ teaspoon baking soda
½ teaspoon salt
1½ cups rolled oats
½ cup flaked coconut

1. Preheat oven to 350°F. In a large bowl, beat brown sugar and butter with an electric mixer on medium speed until light and fluffy. Beat in egg, pineapple with its juice, and rum extract until well blended.

2. Add flour mixed with baking powder, baking soda, and salt and beat until well blended. Stir in oatmeal and coconut.

3. Drop by teaspoonfuls onto greased cookie sheets. Bake 15 to 20 minutes. Let cookies cool on sheets 2 minutes, then remove to a rack and let cool completely.

36 RUM DROPS
Prep: 10 minutes   Bake: 6 to 8 minutes   Makes: about 36

4 tablespoons butter, softened
¼ cup sugar
1 egg

3 tablespoons rum
¾ cup cake flour
½ cup powdered sugar

1. Preheat oven to 350°F. In a medium bowl, beat butter and sugar with an electric mixer on medium speed until well blended. Beat in egg and 2 tablespoons rum. Beat in flour until a soft dough forms, scraping down side of bowl frequently with a rubber spatula.

2. Drop by slightly rounded measuring teaspoonfuls 2 inches apart onto well-greased cookie sheets. Bake 6 to 8 minutes, or until golden brown at edges.

3. Meanwhile, in a small bowl, stir together powdered sugar with remaining 1 tablespoon rum until glaze is smooth. Remove drops from oven and let cool 2 minutes on sheets, then remove to racks. Spread rum glaze over cookies and let cool completely. Store in a tightly covered container.

37 TIC-TAC-TOE COOKIES
Prep: 10 minutes   Bake: 10 to 12 minutes   Makes: about 36

Children love placing the candy and nut pieces on these miniature game boards.

1 stick (4 ounces) butter,
  softened
1 cup firmly packed brown
  sugar
1 egg
1 teaspoon vanilla extract
2¼ cups flour

1 teaspoon baking soda
1 teaspoon cream of tartar
½ teaspoon salt
Miniature chocolate chips or
  candy-coated chocolate
  pieces, such as M&M's
Pecans, cut into tiny pieces

1. Preheat oven to 350°F. In a large bowl, beat butter and brown sugar with an electric mixer on medium speed until well blended. Beat in egg and vanilla until light and fluffy.

2. Mix together flour, soda, cream of tartar, and salt. Add to butter mixture and beat until dough is smooth, scraping down side of bowl frequently with a rubber spatula.

3. Drop by heaping teaspoonfuls 2 inches apart onto lightly greased cookie sheets. Pat to flatten top surface. Press floured tines of a 2-tined kitchen fork into dough to create tic-tac-toe board. Place candies and nuts on board to represent Os and Xs.

4. Bake 10 to 12 minutes, or until golden brown. Let cookies cool 2 minutes on sheets, then remove to racks and let cool completely. Store in a tightly covered container.

38 TROPICAL ISLE COOKIES
Prep: 10 minutes   Bake: 15 to 18 minutes   Makes: about 60

For a more sophisticated version of these tropical treats, substitute rum for the pineapple juice in the glaze.

½ cup granulated sugar
6 tablespoons pineapple
  preserves
6 tablespoons butter
2 eggs
1 teaspoon rum extract

2 cups cake flour
½ teaspoon baking powder
½ teaspoon salt
½ cup flaked coconut
1 cup powdered sugar
2 tablespoons pineapple juice

1. Preheat oven to 350°F. In a large bowl, beat sugar, preserves, and butter with an electric mixer on medium speed until light and fluffy. Beat in eggs and rum extract until well blended.

2. Add cake flour mixed with baking powder and salt and beat until well blended. Stir in coconut.

3. Drop by teaspoonfuls onto greased cookie sheets. Bake 15 to 18 minutes, until edges are light brown. Let cookies cool on sheets 2 minutes, then remove to a rack and let cool completely.

4. In a small bowl, stir together powdered sugar and pineapple juice until blended and smooth. Spread glaze over cooled cookies.

---

39 WHITE CHOCOLATE CHUNK BROWNIE COOKIES

Prep: 15 minutes   Bake: 8 to 10 minutes   Makes: about 42

This rich cookie is adapted from a recipe given to us by our friend Chris Koury, food editor of *Parents Magazine*.

6 tablespoons butter, softened	½ teaspoon instant coffee
½ cup granulated sugar	powder dissolved in
¼ cup firmly packed dark	1 teaspoon water
brown sugar	½ teaspoon vanilla extract
2 (1-ounce) squares	1¼ cups flour
unsweetened chocolate,	½ teaspoon baking soda
melted	¼ teaspoon salt
1 egg, lightly beaten	1 cup white chocolate chunks

1. Preheat oven to 375°F. In a medium bowl, beat butter, granulated sugar, and brown sugar with an electric mixer on medium speed until creamy. Stir in melted chocolate and egg until blended. Add dissolved coffee and vanilla and stir until blended. Beat in flour, baking soda, and salt. Stir in chunks.

2. Drop by teaspoonfuls 1 inch apart onto greased cookie sheets. Bake 8 to 10 minutes, or until set. Let cookies cool 2 minutes on sheets, then remove to a rack and let cool completely.

40 ROCKY ROAD COOKIES

Prep: 10 minutes   Bake: 12 minutes   Makes: about 30

Just like the candy they are named after, these treats overflow with peanuts, chocolate, and marshmallows.

1 stick (4 ounces) butter, softened
¼ cup firmly packed dark brown sugar
1 egg
1 teaspoon vanilla extract
1¼ cups flour
½ teaspoon baking powder
¼ teaspoon salt
½ cup currants
½ cup chopped peanuts
½ cup semisweet chocolate chips
½ cup miniature marshmallows

1. Preheat oven to 375°F. In a medium bowl, beat butter and brown sugar with an electric mixer on medium speed until light and fluffy. Beat in egg and vanilla.

2. Add flour, baking powder, and salt and beat until blended. Stir in currants, peanuts, and chocolate chips.

3. Drop by teaspoonfuls 2 inches apart onto greased cookie sheets. Bake 10 minutes. Remove from oven; leave oven on.

4. Lightly press 1 or 2 marshmallows into center of each cookie. Return to oven and bake 2 minutes, or until golden. Let cookies cool on sheets 2 minutes, then remove to a rack and let cool completely.

Chapter 2

Rolling in Dough

Many people shy away from rolled cookies because they feel it is too hard to roll out and cut the dough. The secret to baking perfect rolled cookies lies in a properly chilled dough and quick handling. Many rolled cookie doughs are stiff enough to be handled right after mixing, while others need to be chilled 2 to 3 hours. This chilling time means that you can't eat them within 20 minutes of deciding to bake. However, it offers the added convenience of mixing up several cookie doughs on one day, refrigerating and baking them the next day, or freezing them and baking within 6 months. This is particularly helpful at holiday times.

We found that rolling out cookies between sheets of wax paper was the most convenient method for us. It provided little flour mess and the wax paper provided support when moving and handling the dough. Sometimes we rolled out the dough between wax paper sheets before chilling it, then stacked the layers of wax paper-encased dough on a cookie sheet and placed them in the refrigerator for several hours or in the freezer for 10 to 20 minutes.

Once chilled, it is easy to cut the dough, peel the cookies off the wax paper, and place them on prepared cookie sheets. Handling rolled cookie dough also varies with the weather. It is much easier to roll out cookie dough on a cool, dry day than on a hot, humid one. Although not all of the recipes mention it, if you have trouble with your dough becoming too soft during hot weather or in a hot kitchen, any of the doughs in this chapter can be placed in the refrigerator or freezer at any stage of rolling, until they are manageable again.

There are many kinds of rolling pins on the market. We found it most efficient to use a heavy pin with a rolling surface that moved around stable handles. Although some of the recipes were tested with a single-piece European pin, we found that it took a lot more experience to roll the dough evenly, and on busy baking days, this type of rolling pin often produced sore fingers. Other choices include a marble pin, a clear glass pin that can be filled with ice water, and a pin that has an automatic thickness guide. Select the one you like best and give rolled cookies a try. With proper handling, they are not difficult, and nothing beats the festive appearance of rolled cookies cut into special shapes and topped with the sparkle of colored sugar. In a pinch, if you don't have a rolling pin, just use a straight-sided soda or mineral water bottle (preferably full and chilled).

41 APRICOT PILLOWS

Prep: 10 minutes   Chill: 2 to 3 hours
Bake: 10 to 12 minutes   Makes: about 20

½ cup sugar
1 stick (4 ounces) butter, softened
1 egg
½ teaspoon almond extract
1½ cups flour

½ teaspoon baking powder
⅛ teaspoon salt
¼ cup firmly packed dried apricots (6 whole or 12 half apricots)
1 tablespoon honey

1. In a medium bowl, beat sugar and butter with an electric mixer on medium speed until well blended. Beat in egg and almond extract until light and fluffy.

2. Mix together flour, baking powder, and salt and add, beating on low speed until dough is smooth, scraping down side of bowl frequently with a rubber spatula. Wrap and refrigerate dough 2 to 3 hours, until firm.

3. Meanwhile, finely chop dried apricots. In a small bowl, stir together apricots and honey. Set apricot filling aside at room temperature until dough has chilled.

4. Preheat oven to 350°F. Between pieces of wax paper, roll out dough ⅛ inch thick. Cut out cookies with 2-inch round cutters. Reroll scraps to make additional cookies.

5. Place half of cookies 2 inches apart on lightly greased cookie sheets. Spoon about ½ teaspoon apricot filling onto center of cookies. Moisten edges of cookies and top with remaining cookies to make a sandwich. Press edges together with fingertips to seal. Pierce center of each "pillow" with tines of a fork.

6. Bake 10 to 12 minutes, or until edges are golden brown. Let cookies cool 2 minutes on sheets, then remove to racks and let cool completely. Store in a tightly covered container.

42 CARDAMOM COOKIES

Prep: 10 minutes   Bake: 8 to 10 minutes   Makes: about 24

Cardamom brings an exotic flair to these crisp butter cookies.

½ cup sugar
1 stick (4 ounces) butter, softened
1¾ cups cake flour

1 tablespoon ground cardamom
⅛ teaspoon salt
¼ cup sliced natural almonds

1. Preheat oven to 350°F. Reserve 1 tablespoon sugar. In a medium bowl, beat butter and remaining sugar with an electric mixer on medium speed until well blended. Beat in flour mixed with cardamom and salt. Form dough into a ball.

2. Between pieces of floured wax paper, roll out dough ⅛ inch thick. Cut into cookies with a 2½-inch round cutter. Reroll scraps to make additional cookies.

3. Place cookies 2 inches apart on lightly greased cookie sheets. Sprinkle reserved sugar and sliced almonds on top.

4. Bake 8 to 10 minutes, or until edges are golden brown. Let cookies cool 2 minutes on sheets, then remove to racks and let cool completely. Store in a tightly covered container.

---

43 BANBURY TARTS
Prep: 10 minutes   Chill: 30 minutes
Bake: 18 to 20 minutes   Makes: 16

1 stick (4 ounces) butter, softened	¼ teaspoon salt
1¼ cups sugar	1½ cups muscat raisins or regular raisins
2 eggs	⅓ cup lemon juice
2 teaspoons vanilla extract	2 teaspoons grated lemon zest
1½ cups flour	1 tablespoon cracker or bread crumbs
½ teaspoon baking powder	

1. In a medium bowl, beat butter and ¼ cup sugar with an electric mixer on medium speed until well blended. Beat in 1 egg and vanilla until light and fluffy.

2. Add flour mixed with baking powder and salt and beat on low speed until a stiff dough forms, scraping down side of bowl frequently with a rubber spatula. Wrap and refrigerate dough at least 30 minutes, or until firm.

3. Meanwhile, in a medium bowl, combine raisins, remaining 1 cup sugar, remaining egg, lemon juice, lemon zest, and cracker crumbs. Stir to mix well.

4. Preheat oven to 350°F. Between pieces of wax paper, roll out half of dough ¼ inch thick to make a 9-inch square. Repeat with remaining piece of dough to make another 9-inch square. Peel wax paper from top of one square of dough. Using bottom paper for support, invert dough square into a lightly greased 9-inch square pan; peel off and discard wax paper.

5. Spoon raisin filling onto pastry in pan; top with remaining pastry square. Lightly score top of dough with point of knife to make 16 squares. Poke a hole in center of each square.

6. Bake pan of tarts 18 to 20 minutes, or until cookie crust is golden and filling is bubbly. Remove to a rack and let cool completely in pan. Cut into 16 squares where scored and store in a tightly covered container.

44 CHEESE SAVORIES

Prep: 10 minutes   Chill: 30 minutes   Bake: 8 to 10 minutes
Makes: 36

These tasty little cheese biscuits are the perfect accompaniment to drinks before dinner.

⅓ cup coarsely grated
  Parmesan cheese
1 stick (4 ounces) butter,
  softened

1½ cups flour
½ teaspoon baking powder
¼ teaspoon cayenne

1. Set aside 2 tablespoons of grated cheese. In a medium bowl, beat butter and remaining cheese with an electric mixer on medium speed until well blended. Add flour mixed with baking powder and cayenne and beat on low speed until dough is smooth, scraping down sides of bowl frequently with a rubber scraper. Wrap and refrigerate dough at least 30 minutes, or until firm.

2. Preheat oven to 350°F. Between pieces of wax paper, roll out dough ¼ inch thick. Cut out rounds with 2-inch cookie cutters. Reroll scraps to make additional savories.

3. Place savories 2 inches apart on lightly greased cookie sheets. Sprinkle reserved cheese on top. Bake 8 to 10 minutes, or until edges are golden brown. Let savories cool 2 minutes on sheets, then remove to racks and let cool completely. Store in a tightly covered container.

45 CHOCOLATE SANDWICH COOKIES

Prep: 10 minutes   Chill: 2 hours   Bake: 10 to 12 minutes
Makes: about 16

1 stick (4 ounces) plus
  2 tablespoons butter,
  softened
¾ cup granulated sugar
1 egg
1½ teaspoons vanilla extract
1¾ cups flour

¼ cup unsweetened cocoa
  powder
⅛ teaspoon salt
1½ cups powdered sugar
2 to 3 teaspoons milk
1 (1-ounce) square semisweet
  chocolate, melted

1. In a large bowl, beat 1 stick butter and granulated sugar with an electric mixer on medium speed until well blended. Beat in egg and 1 teaspoon vanilla until light and fluffy.

2. On low speed, beat in flour, cocoa powder, and salt until dough is smooth, scraping down side of bowl frequently with a rubber spatula. Wrap and refrigerate dough 2 to 3 hours, until firm.

3. Preheat oven to 350°F. Between sheets of wax paper, roll out dough ⅛ inch thick. Cut out cookies with a 2-inch round cutter. Reroll scraps to make additional cookies. If rolled dough is difficult to handle, place in freezer 15 to 20 minutes before cutting.

4. Arrange cookies 2 inches apart on lightly greased cookie sheets. Bake 10 to 12 minutes, or until cookies are firm. Let cookies cool 2 minutes on sheets, then remove to racks and let cool completely.

5. Meanwhile, in a small bowl, with an electric mixer on high speed, beat remaining 2 tablespoons butter with powdered sugar, remaining ½ teaspoon vanilla, and enough milk to make a spreadable frosting.

6. Spread frosting onto flat bottom sides of half of cookies. Top with remaining cookies, flat sides toward filling. Drizzle melted chocolate over chocolate cookie sandwiches. Set on wire rack to cool completely.

---

46 FIG BARS
Prep: 10 minutes   Chill: 30 minutes   Bake: 20 to 25 minutes
Makes: 24

These are as close as we could come to those favorite fig bars you buy in the store that have the same last name as Sir Isaac Newton.

1 **stick (4 ounces) butter, softened**	⅛ **teaspoon salt**
⅓ **cup sugar**	8 **ounces dried figs**
1 **egg**	¼ **cup natural almonds**
½ **teaspoon vanilla extract**	¼ **cup apricot preserves**
1½ **cups flour**	1 **tablespoon lemon juice**
¼ **teaspoon baking powder**	2 **teaspoons grated lemon zest**
¼ **teaspoon grated nutmeg**	¼ **teaspoon cinnamon**

1. In a medium bowl, beat butter and sugar with an electric mixer on medium speed until well blended. Beat in egg and vanilla until light and fluffy.

2. Add flour, baking powder, nutmeg, and salt and beat on low speed until dough is smooth, scraping down side of bowl frequently with a rubber spatula. Divide dough in half. Wrap and refrigerate both pieces of dough at least 30 minutes, or until firm enough to handle.

3. Meanwhile, in a food processor, combine dried figs, almonds, apricot preserves, lemon juice, lemon zest, and cinnamon. Process until finely chopped. Set fig filling aside.

4. Preheat oven to 350°F. Between pieces of wax paper, roll out half of dough to make a 12 × 6-inch rectangle about ¼ inch thick. Spoon half of fig filling in a 2-inch strip down length of dough rectangle. Lift sides of dough over filling and overlap; pinch to seal. Repeat with remaining half of dough and filling.

5. Place rolls, seam side down, on lightly greased baking sheet. Pinch ends shut. Bake 20 to 25 minutes, or until edges of rolls are golden brown. Let cool 2 minutes on sheets, then remove to racks and let cool completely. Cut each roll into 12 bars. Store in a tightly covered container.

47 CINNAMON BOW TIE COOKIES
Prep: 15 minutes   Bake: 10 minutes   Makes: 24

Bonnie re-created these not-too-sweet cookies her Grandma Mary used to make out of the scraps from her day's baking.

¾ to 1 cup flour
¼ cup plus 1 tablespoon sugar
¾ teaspoon baking powder
½ teaspoon lemon zest
½ teaspoon orange zest
  Pinch of salt

2 tablespoons vegetable oil
1 egg
1½ teaspoons fresh lemon
  juice
1 tablespoon orange juice
¼ teaspoon cinnamon

1. Preheat oven to 350°F. In a medium bowl, mix ¾ cup flour and ¼ cup sugar with baking powder, lemon zest, orange zest, and salt. Beat with a wooden spoon until blended. Mix in oil, egg, lemon juice, and orange juice just until dough forms. Stir in enough remaining flour so dough is not sticky.

2. Stir together remaining 1 tablespoon sugar and cinnamon. On well-floured board, roll dough to a 12 × 8-inch rectangle. Sprinkle with cinnamon sugar. Cut in half lengthwise, then into 1-inch strips, making 24 rectangles about 4 × 1 inch. Twist in center to make bow tie. Place on a greased cookie sheet.

3. Bake 10 minutes, or until golden. Remove to a rack and let cool completely.

48 LEMON SANDWICH COOKIES
Prep: 10 minutes   Chill: 2 hours   Bake: 10 to 12 minutes
Makes: about 16

Refreshingly lemony, these are delicious even without the white chocolate coating.

1 stick (4 ounces) plus
  2 tablespoons butter,
  softened
¾ cup granulated sugar
1 egg
1 teaspoon vanilla extract
1½ teaspoons grated lemon zest

2 cups flour
⅛ teaspoon salt
1½ cups powdered sugar
2 to 3 teaspoons lemon juice
3 ounces white chocolate,
  melted (optional)

1. In a large bowl, beat 1 stick butter and granulated sugar with an electric mixer on medium speed until well blended. Beat in egg, vanilla, and 1 teaspoon lemon zest until light and fluffy.

2. On low speed, beat in flour and salt until dough is smooth, scraping down side of bowl frequently with a rubber spatula. Wrap and refrigerate dough 2 to 3 hours, until firm.

3. Preheat oven to 350°F. Between pieces of wax paper, roll out dough ⅛ inch thick. Cut out cookies with a 2-inch round cutter. Reroll scraps to make additional cookies. If rolled dough is difficult to handle, place in freezer 15 to 20 minutes before cutting.

4. Arrange cookies 2 inches apart on lightly greased cookie sheets. Bake 10 to 12 minutes, or until edges are golden brown. Let cookies cool 2 minutes on sheets, then remove to racks and let cool completely.

5. Meanwhile, in a small bowl, with an electric mixer on high speed, beat remaining 2 tablespoons butter and ½ teaspoon lemon zest with powdered sugar and enough lemon juice to make a spreadable frosting.

6. Spread frosting over flat bottom sides of half of cookies. Top with remaining cookies, flat sides toward filling. If desired, dip tops of cookies into melted white chocolate. Set on wire rack over sheets of wax paper to cool.

49 CLOVE COOKIES
Prep: 10 minutes   Bake: 10 to 12 minutes   Makes: about 40

Although most people will want to discard the whole cloves before eating these cookies, they add a signature design to the buttery bites.

1½ sticks (6 ounces) butter, softened	2 cups flour
½ cup sugar	½ teaspoon baking powder
1 egg	½ teaspoon ground cloves
1 teaspoon vanilla extract	⅛ teaspoon salt
	About 40 whole cloves

1. Preheat oven to 350°F. In a medium bowl, beat butter and sugar with an electric mixer on medium speed until well blended. Beat in egg and vanilla until light and fluffy.

2. Beat in flour, baking powder, ground cloves, and salt on low speed until dough is smooth, scraping down side of bowl frequently with a rubber spatula.

3. Between pieces of floured wax paper, roll out dough ¼ inch thick. Cut out cookies with a 2-inch round cutter. Reroll scraps to make additional cookies.

4. Place cookies 2 inches apart on lightly greased cookie sheets. Press a whole clove into top of each cookie. Bake 10 to 12 minutes, or until edges are golden brown. Let cookies cool 2 minutes on sheets, then remove to racks and let cool completely. Store in a tightly covered container.

50 CRISP GINGER COOKIES
Prep: 10 minutes   Chill: 2 hours   Bake: 10 to 12 minutes
Makes: about 32

Bonnie's friend Nancy Bostwick makes these cookies every Christmas. They are light and crisp and can be made in a jiffy.

½ **cup solid vegetable shortening**	1 **teaspoon cinnamon**
½ **cup sugar**	½ **teaspoon ground ginger**
½ **cup dark molasses**	½ **teaspoon baking soda**
1¾ **cups flour**	¼ **teaspoon salt**

1. In a medium bowl, beat shortening, ½ cup sugar, and molasses with an electric mixer on medium speed until well blended.

2. On low speed, beat in flour mixed with cinnamon, ginger, baking soda, and salt. Beat until dough is smooth, scraping down side of bowl frequently with a rubber spatula. Wrap and refrigerate dough 2 to 3 hours, until firm.

3. Preheat oven to 350°F. Between pieces of wax paper, roll out dough ¼ inch thick. Cut into 2-inch squares. Reroll scraps to make additional cookies. Arrange cookies 2 inches apart on lightly greased cookie sheets.

4. Bake 10 to 12 minutes, or until edges brown. Let cookies cool 2 minutes on sheets, then remove to racks and let cool completely. Store in a tightly covered container.

51 PATCHWORK COOKIES
Prep: 10 minutes   Chill: 10 minutes   Bake: 10 to 12 minutes
Makes: 36

1 **stick (4 ounces) butter, softened**	1½ **cups flour**
½ **cup sugar**	¼ **teaspoon baking powder**
1 **egg**	⅛ **teaspoon salt**
2 **teaspoons vanilla extract**	**Yellow, red, blue, and green food coloring**

1. In a medium bowl, beat butter and sugar with an electric mixer on medium speed until well blended. Beat in egg and vanilla until light and fluffy. Add flour mixed with baking powder and salt and beat on low speed until dough is smooth, scraping down side of bowl frequently with a rubber spatula.

2. Divide dough into quarters; place in 4 small bowls. Add 3 drops of yellow food coloring to one bowl, 3 drops red to another, 2 drops blue to another, and 2 drops green to the last. With a clean fork, stir color into each batch of dough until evenly blended.

3. Break each colored ball of dough into 8 to 10 pieces. On a sheet of wax paper, arrange pieces of assorted dough so that colors are randomly scattered. Pat pieces together. Cover dough with another sheet of wax paper and roll into a 12-inch square. Place on a cookie sheet and set in freezer for 10 to 15 minutes, or until firm.

4. Preheat oven to 350°F. Peel off top piece of wax paper. With a sharp knife or a fluted pastry cutter, make 5 cuts in each direction to divide dough into 36 (2-inch) squares. Place squares 2 inches apart on lightly greased cookie sheets.

5. Bake 10 to 12 minutes, or until edges are golden brown. Let cookies cool 2 minutes on sheets, then remove to racks and let cool completely. Store in a tightly covered container.

---

52 PEANUT BUTTER AND JELLY COOKIE SANDWICHES

Prep: 10 minutes   Chill: 1 hour   Bake: 10 to 12 minutes
Makes: about 24

The classic combination of peanut butter and jelly makes a delicious and easy cookie filling.

1 **stick (4 ounces) butter, softened**	2 **cups flour**
¾ **cup sugar**	¼ **teaspoon grated nutmeg**
1 **egg**	⅛ **teaspoon salt**
1 **teaspoon vanilla extract**	¼ **cup red raspberry jelly**
	¼ **cup smooth peanut butter**

1. In a large bowl, beat butter and sugar with an electric mixer on medium speed until well blended. Beat in egg and vanilla until light and fluffy.

2. Add flour, nutmeg, and salt and beat on low speed until dough is smooth, scraping down side of bowl frequently with a rubber spatula. Wrap and refrigerate dough 1 hour, until firm.

3. Preheat oven to 350°F. Between pieces of wax paper, roll out dough ⅛ inch thick. Cut out cookies with a 2-inch round cutter. Reroll scraps to make additional cookies. If rolled dough is difficult to handle, place in freezer 15 to 20 minutes to firm up.

4. Place cookies 2 inches apart on lightly greased cookie sheets. Bake 10 to 12 minutes, or until edges are golden brown. Let cookies cool 2 minutes on sheets, then remove to racks and let cool completely.

5. Spread flat bottom sides of half of cookies with jelly. Spread flat bottoms of remaining half with peanut butter. Press cookies together to make sandwiches. Store in a tightly covered container.

53 ROLLED SUGAR COOKIES

Prep: 10 minutes   Chill: 2 hours   Bake: 10 to 12 minutes
Makes: about 36

These basic rolled sugar cookies can be dressed up for any holiday, depending upon the cookie cutters you choose. They can also be topped before baking with colored sugar or candy sprinkles.

⅔ cup sugar
1 stick (4 ounces) butter, softened
1 egg

1 teaspoon vanilla extract
1½ cups flour
½ teaspoon baking powder
⅛ teaspoon salt

1. In a medium bowl, beat sugar and butter with an electric mixer on medium speed until well blended. Beat in egg and vanilla until light and fluffy.

2. On low speed, beat in flour mixed with baking powder and salt until dough is smooth, scraping down side of bowl frequently with a rubber spatula. Wrap and refrigerate dough 2 to 3 hours, until firm.

3. Preheat oven to 350°F. Between pieces of wax paper, roll out dough ¼ inch thick. Cut out cookies with 2-inch cutters. Reroll scraps to make additional cookies.

4. Arrange cookies 2 inches apart on lightly greased cookie sheets. Bake 10 to 12 minutes, or until edges are golden brown. Let cookies cool 2 minutes on sheets, then remove to racks and let cool completely. Store in a tightly covered container.

---

54 RICOTTA CHEESE COOKIES

Prep: 20 minutes   Chill: 2 hours   Bake: 12 to 15 minutes
Makes: 30

These traditional Italian cookies are designed to be baked and served on the same day. They do not store well.

1 stick (4 ounces) butter, softened
⅓ cup ricotta cheese
2 tablespoons granulated sugar

½ teaspoon vanilla extract
1⅓ cups flour
3 to 4 tablespoons seedless red raspberry preserves
Powdered sugar

1. In a medium bowl, beat butter, ricotta cheese, granulated sugar, and vanilla with an electric mixer on medium speed until well blended.

2. Beat in flour on low speed just until dough is smooth, scraping down side of bowl frequently with a rubber spatula. (Do not overbeat or dough will toughen.) Divide dough in half. Wrap tightly and refrigerate 2 to 3 hours, or until firm.

3. Preheat oven to 400°F. Between pieces of wax paper, roll out each half of dough to make a 10 × 6-inch rectangle. Cut each rectangle into 15 (2-inch) squares. Dab a heaping ¼ teaspoon of preserves onto each dough square. Fold 1 corner of dough diagonally over preserves to make a triangle; press edges together to seal.

4. Place triangles 2 inches apart on lightly greased cookie sheets. Bake 12 to 15 minutes, or until edges are golden brown. Let cookies cool 2 minutes on sheets, then remove to racks to cool completely. Sift some powdered sugar over cookies just before serving.

---

55 PINWHEEL COOKIES
Prep: 20 minutes   Chill: 3 hours   Bake: 8 to 10 minutes
Makes: about 48

These chocolate lemon spirals make any cookie plate spectacular.

2¼ cups flour
½ teaspoon baking soda
½ teaspoon salt
1 stick (4 ounces) butter, softened
1 cup sugar

2 eggs, at room temperature
1 teaspoon vanilla extract
1 (1-ounce) square unsweetened baking chocolate, melted
1 teaspoon lemon extract

1. In a small bowl, combine flour, baking soda, and salt. Stir or whisk gently to blend.

2. In a medium bowl, with an electric mixer on medium speed, beat butter and sugar until light and fluffy. Beat in eggs and vanilla.

3. Add flour to butter-sugar mixture and blend well. Divide dough in half between 2 bowls. Stir chocolate into one half; stir lemon extract into the other. Cover each bowl and refrigerate at least 1 hour, until firm.

4. Roll out each piece of dough between 2 pieces of wax paper into an 8 × 12-inch rectangle. Place 1 rectangle on top of the other and roll up from a long side into a 12-inch roll. Wrap in wax paper and refrigerate until firm, at least 2 hours.

5. Preheat oven to 350°F. Using a sharp knife, cut dough into ¼-inch slices. Arrange about 3 inches apart on ungreased baking sheets. Bake 8 to 10 minutes, until lightly browned. Let stand 5 minutes, then remove to a rack and let cool completely.

56   FRENCH SUGAR CRACKERS
Prep: 10 minutes   Chill: 2 hours   Bake: 8 to 10 minutes   Makes: 32

The perfect accompaniment for afternoon tea.

½ cup sugar	½ teaspoon vanilla extract
1 stick (4 ounces) butter, softened	1 cup flour
	¼ teaspoon salt
1 egg, separated	¼ cup finely chopped walnuts

1. Set aside 1 tablespoon sugar. In a large bowl, beat butter and remaining sugar with an electric mixer on medium speed until well blended. Beat egg yolk and vanilla into butter mixture until light and fluffy.

2. Beat in flour and salt until dough is smooth, scraping down side of bowl frequently with a rubber spatula. Wrap and refrigerate dough until it is firm, at least 2 hours.

3. When ready to bake crackers, preheat oven to 350°F. With a floured rolling pin, roll out half of dough on a lightly greased cookie sheet to make an 8-inch square. With a knife or a fluted pastry wheel, even edges of dough. Cut dough into sixteen 2-inch squares. Repeat with second half of dough. Beat egg white until frothy. Brush white over dough and sprinkle with nuts and reserved 1 tablespoon sugar.

4. Bake 8 to 10 minutes, or until firm and very lightly browned on edges. Separate crackers slightly where cut. Let cool 5 minutes, then transfer crackers to a rack and let cool completely. Store in a tightly covered container.

57   WALNUT SAVORIES
Prep: 10 minutes   Chill: 30 minutes   Bake: 8 to 10 minutes
Makes: about 36

Serve a plate of these savory cookies with wine and apples for informal entertaining.

1 egg, lightly beaten	¼ teaspoon salt
1 stick (4 ounces) butter, softened	¼ teaspoon cracked black pepper
1½ cups flour	2 tablespoons finely chopped walnuts
½ teaspoon baking powder	
¼ teaspoon thyme	

1. Set aside 1 tablespoon of egg in a custard cup. In a medium bowl, beat butter and remaining egg with an electric mixer on medium speed until well blended. Add flour mixed with baking powder, thyme, salt, and pepper and beat on low speed until dough is smooth, scraping down side of bowl frequently with a rubber spatula. Wrap and refrigerate dough at least 30 minutes, or until firm.

2. Preheat oven to 350°F. Between pieces of wax paper, roll out dough ¼ inch thick. Cut out rounds with 2-inch cookie cutters. Reroll scraps to make additional savories.

3. Place savories 2 inches apart on lightly greased cookie sheets. Brush tops with reserved egg and sprinkle walnuts on top. Bake 8 to 10 minutes, or until edges are golden brown. Let savories cool 2 minutes on sheets, then remove to racks and let cool completely. Store in a tightly covered container.

---

58   SUGAR 'N' SPICE COOKIES
Prep: 10 minutes   Bake: 12 to 15 minutes   Makes: 16

Even on a busy night, you can surprise your family with these easy, aromatic cookies, warm from the oven.

⅔ cup sugar	1 teaspoon cinnamon
1 stick (4 ounces) butter, softened	½ teaspoon baking powder
	½ teaspoon ground ginger
1 egg	¼ teaspoon grated nutmeg
1 teaspoon vanilla extract	¼ teaspoon ground allspice
1½ cups flour	⅛ teaspoon salt

1. Preheat oven to 350°F. Set aside 2 teaspoons sugar. In a medium bowl, beat butter and remaining sugar with an electric mixer on medium speed until well blended. Beat in egg and vanilla until light and fluffy.

2. Add flour mixed with cinnamon, baking powder, ginger, nutmeg, allspice, and salt. Beat on low speed until a stiff dough forms, scraping down side of bowl frequently with a rubber spatula.

3. Divide dough in half. On a lightly greased cookie sheet, roll out half of dough with a floured rolling pin to make an 8-inch round. Score round into 8 wedges. Repeat with remaining dough on another cookie sheet. Sprinkle 1 teaspoon reserved sugar over each round of dough.

4. Bake rounds 12 to 15 minutes, or until edges are golden brown. Let cookies cool 2 minutes on sheets, then remove to racks and let cool completely. To serve, break into wedges. Store in a tightly covered container.

59   HONEY BRAN CRISPS
Prep: 10 minutes   Chill: 1 hour   Bake: 7 to 9 minutes
Makes: about 60

Here's a crisp, not-too-sweet cookie, perfect for teatime.

2 cups flour
1 teaspoon baking powder
1½ teaspoons cinnamon
½ teaspoon salt
1 stick (4 ounces) butter,
   softened

½ cup honey
½ teaspoon vanilla extract
1 cup bran flakes cereal,
   slightly crushed
½ cup powdered sugar

1. In a small bowl, combine flour, baking powder, cinnamon, and salt. Stir or whisk gently to blend.

2. In a medium bowl, beat butter and honey with an electric mixer on medium speed until light and fluffy. Beat in vanilla.

3. Add flour mixture and beat until blended. Stir in cereal. Cover with wax paper and refrigerate dough about 1 hour, or until firm.

4. Preheat oven to 350°F. Roll dough between 2 sheets of wax paper to ⅛-inch thickness. Cut out rounds using a 2-inch cookie cutter dipped in flour. Place cookies 2 inches apart on greased cookie sheets. Bake 7 to 9 minutes, or until edges just begin to turn golden brown. Remove to rack to cool completely. When cool, dust tops with powdered sugar.

60   LEMON SHORTBREAD COOKIES
Prep: 5 minutes   Bake: 20 to 25 minutes   Makes: about 20

1 stick (4 ounces) butter,
   softened
¼ cup firmly packed dark
   brown sugar
2 teaspoons grated lemon zest

½ teaspoon lemon extract
¼ teaspoon vanilla extract
1 cup flour
¼ teaspoon salt

1. Preheat oven to 325°F. In a medium bowl, beat butter and brown sugar with an electric mixer on medium speed until light and fluffy. Beat in lemon zest, lemon extract, and vanilla.

2. Add flour and salt to butter-sugar mixture and blend well. With a rolling pin on a lightly floured surface, roll out dough ¼ inch thick. Cut out cookies using a 2-inch round cutter and place 2 inches apart on ungreased cookie sheets. Reroll scraps.

3. Bake 20 to 25 minutes, until cookies are pale golden, not brown. Let stand 2 minutes. Remove to a rack and let cool completely.

61 OATMEAL SHORTBREAD

Prep: 10 minutes   Bake: 12 to 15 minutes   Makes: 16

This quick recipe can be rolled into rounds, cut into wedges, and baked to buttery perfection in no time.

1 stick (4 ounces) butter, softened	¾ cup flour
⅓ cup firmly packed brown sugar	½ cup rolled oats
1 teaspoon vanilla extract	1 teaspoon cinnamon
	⅛ teaspoon salt

1. Preheat oven to 350°F. In a medium bowl, beat butter, brown sugar, and vanilla with an electric mixer on medium speed until well blended.

2. Add flour, oatmeal, cinnamon, and salt and beat on low speed until a stiff dough forms, scraping down side of bowl frequently with a rubber spatula.

3. Divide dough in half. On a lightly greased cookie sheet, roll out one half of dough with a floured rolling pin to make an 8-inch round. Score round into 8 wedges. Repeat with remaining dough on a second cookie sheet.

4. Bake rounds 12 to 15 minutes, or until edges are golden brown. Let cool 2 minutes on sheets, then remove to racks and let cool completely. To serve, break into wedges where scored. Store in a tightly covered container.

Chapter 3

In Great Shape

Shaped cookies vary in difficulty from simple hand-rolled balls to fancy pressed spritz cookies. They offer the opportunity for the ultimate creativity and the tactile joy of molding something wonderful by hand. Children love making shaped cookies. They are even more fun than playing with clay because the results make a delicious snack.

The dough for shaped cookies is usually a bit stiffer than that for dropped cookies and not quite as stiff as that for rolled or refrigerator cookies. When it is the perfect consistency, you should be able to mold it by hand at room temperature with no trouble. If the dough is too sticky, either oiling or flouring the hands will make it easier to shape the dough. If the dough is too crumbly, moistening the hands will make the job easier. If your drop cookie dough turns out too dry or your rolled or refrigerator cookie dough too sticky, shaped cookies come to the rescue. You can roll the dough into balls or pat it into flat rounds on a cookie sheet and invent a new kind of cookie.

When shaping cookies, it is important to work quickly so that the heat of your hands does not melt the butter in the dough. Most shaped cookies are slightly higher in fat than some other varieties in order to make them more manageable; however, this also makes them more susceptible to softening in warm weather and when exposed to the heat of hands for too long.

In preparation for busy holiday seasons, shaped cookies can be molded ahead and frozen on cookie sheets until hard, then transferrd to freezer containers. Shortly before serving, place the formed cookies on cookie sheets and bake. Guests will be delighted by the warm-from-the-oven cookies and impressed that you took the time to make them.

Spritz cookies are special at any season. When preparing spritz cookie dough, it is important not to include any chopped fruit or nuts that would catch in the opening of the template. It is always important to place cookies on cool cookie sheets, but it is doubly important for spritz cookies, because they are dependent upon the cookies sticking to the tray slightly in order to pull free from the cookie press.

Whether you shape your cookies in one of the traditional forms or sculpt something entirely different, they are sure to let people know that you have taken the time to make something special by hand just to please them.

62   ALMOND BUTTER COOKIES

Prep: 20 minutes   Bake: 12 to 15 minutes   Makes: about 42

Children will love to help roll and shape these cookies.

½ cup plus 2 tablespoons sugar
1 stick (4 ounces) butter, softened
2 eggs
2 tablespoons milk
1 teaspoon vanilla extract

½ teaspoon almond extract
2 cups flour
¼ teaspoon salt
2 tablespoons minced blanched almonds

1. Preheat oven to 350°F. In a large bowl, beat ½ cup sugar and butter with an electric mixer on medium speed until well blended. Separate 1 egg; reserve white. Beat remaining whole egg and egg yolk, milk, vanilla, and almond extract into butter and sugar until light and fluffy.

2. On low speed, beat in flour and salt until dough is smooth, scraping down side of bowl frequently with a rubber spatula.

3. Divide dough into 1-inch balls. With palms of hands, roll each dough ball to make a 5-inch rope. Set ropes 2 inches apart on lightly greased cookie sheets and shape into S's. In a small bowl, whisk egg white until frothy. In a cup, combine remaining 2 tablespoons sugar and minced almonds. Brush S's with egg white. Sprinkle sugar-almond mixture on top.

4. Bake 12 to 15 minutes, or until firm and very lightly browned. Remove cookies to a rack and let cool completely. Store in a tightly covered container.

63   ALMOND CRESCENTS

Prep: 15 minutes   Chill: 1 hour   Bake: 8 to 10 minutes
Makes: about 60

1½ sticks (6 ounces) unsalted butter, softened
1½ cups powdered sugar
1 tablespoon half-and-half

1 teaspoon almond extract
⅛ teaspoon salt
1½ cups flour
½ cup finely chopped almonds

1. In a medium bowl, beat butter and 1 cup powdered sugar with an electric mixer on medium speed until light and fluffy. Beat in half-and-half, almond extract, and salt until well blended.

2. Add flour to butter-sugar mixture and blend well. Stir in almonds. Cover and refrigerate at least 1 hour until firm.

3. Preheat oven to 350°F. Shape dough by teaspoonfuls into crescents, each about 1½ inches long, and place 2 inches apart on greased cookie sheets. Bake 8 to 10 minutes, or until edges just begin to brown. Let cool 5 minutes on sheets, then roll cookies in remaining ½ cup powdered sugar, transfer to a rack, and let cool completely.

64 ALMOND CHEWS
Prep: 10 minutes   Chill: 1 hour   Bake: 8 to 10 minutes
Makes: about 36

1 stick (4 ounces) butter,
softened
½ cup firmly packed brown
sugar
1 cup almond paste (about
8 ounces)
2 tablespoons half-and-half or
milk

1 teaspoon almond extract
½ teaspoon vanilla extract
½ teaspoon salt
¾ cup flour
Slivered almonds

1. In a medium bowl, beat butter and brown sugar with an electric mixer on medium speed until light and fluffy. Beat in almond paste. Add half-and-half, almond extract, vanilla, and salt.

2. Add flour to almond-butter mixture and blend well. Cover and refrigerate at least 1 hour until firm.

3. Preheat oven to 350°F. Shape dough into 1½-inch balls and place 3 inches apart on ungreased cookie sheets. Flatten each ball into a disk and arrange parallel lines of slivered almonds on each one.

4. Bake 8 to 10 minutes, or until edges are just lightly brown. Let cool 4 minutes, then remove to a rack and let cool completely.

65 ALMOND SHORTBREAD
Prep: 5 minutes   Bake: 20 to 25 minutes   Makes: 16

1 stick (4 ounces) butter,
softened
¼ cup firmly packed dark
brown sugar
½ teaspoon almond extract
¼ teaspoon vanilla extract

1 cup flour
½ cup plus 2 tablespoons
finely ground toasted
almonds
¼ teaspoon salt

1. Preheat oven to 325°F. In a medium bowl, beat butter and brown sugar with an electric mixer on medium speed until light and fluffy. Beat in almond extract and vanilla.

2. Add flour, ½ cup ground almonds, and salt and mix until blended. Divide dough in half. Press each half evenly over bottom of a 9-inch pie pan, crimp edges, and prick all over with a fork. Using a knife, cut into 8 wedges each. Sprinkle remaining almonds over dough.

3. Bake 20 to 25 minutes, until pale golden, not brown. Let cool in pan 5 minutes, then recut into wedges, transfer to a wire rack, and let cool completely.

66   ALMOND LOGS
Prep: 20 minutes   Chill: 1 hour   Bake: 8 to 10 minutes   Makes: 48

1 stick (4 ounces) butter,
    softened
4 ounces cream cheese,
    softened
¾ cup granulated sugar
1 egg yolk
½ teaspoon vanilla extract
½ teaspoon almond extract

1½ cups flour
¾ cup finely ground almonds
½ teaspoon baking powder
¼ teaspoon salt
1 cup powdered sugar
2 tablespoons Amaretto
    (almond-flavored liqueur)

1. In a medium bowl, beat butter, cream cheese, and granulated sugar with an electric mixer on medium speed until light and fluffy. Beat in egg yolk, vanilla, and almond extract.

2. Add flour mixed with ¼ cup ground almonds, baking powder, and salt and beat until blended. Cover and refrigerate at least 1 hour, until firm.

3. Preheat oven to 375°F. Divide one fourth of dough into 12 pieces. Roll each piece into a 2½-inch-long log and place logs 1 inch apart on ungreased cookie sheets. Repeat with remaining dough.

4. Bake 8 to 10 minutes, or until edges just begin to turn golden brown. Let cookies cool on sheets 2 minutes, then remove to a rack and let cool completely.

5. In a small bowl, stir together powdered sugar and Amaretto to make an icing of spreading consistency. Dip ends of cooled cookies into icing to coat about one third, then into remaining ½ cup ground almonds.

67   CARAMEL CHOCOLATE OATIES
Prep: 10 minutes   Bake: 8 to 10 minutes   Makes: about 36

1½ sticks (6 ounces) butter,
    softened
½ cup granulated sugar
¼ cup firmly packed dark
    brown sugar
1½ cups rolled oats
¾ cup flour
1 teaspoon baking powder

1 teaspoon grated lemon zest
½ teaspoon salt
¼ teaspoon lemon extract
1 cup semisweet mini
    chocolate chips (6 ounces)
10 caramel candies, finely
    diced

1. Preheat oven to 350°F. In a large bowl, beat butter, granulated sugar, and brown sugar with an electric mixer on medium speed until creamy. Add oatmeal, flour, baking powder, lemon zest, salt, and lemon extract and stir until well blended. Mix in chocolate chips and caramels.

2. Place golf ball–sized rounds 2 inches apart on ungreased cookie sheets. Bake 8 to 10 minutes, until browned at edges. Let stand 5 minutes on cookie sheets, then remove to a wire rack and let cool completely.

68   BLACK-EYED SUSANS
Prep: 10 minutes   Bake: 10 to 12 minutes   Makes: about 36

1   recipe Vanilla Spritz
     Cookies or Chocolate
     Spritz Cookies (pages 66
     or 50)
½   cup semisweet chocolate
     chips, melted

2   tablespoons sour cream
1   tablespoon orange-flavored
     liqueur or 1 teaspoon
     vanilla extract

1. Preheat oven to 350°F. Prepare cookie dough as directed in vanilla or chocolate spritz cookie recipe. Spoon dough into a cookie press fitted with a flower template or a large pastry bag fitted with a large flower tip.

2. Press or pipe cookies 2 inches apart onto lightly greased cookie sheets to form 1½-inch flowers. With thumb, press a level indentation in center, filling any open space with dough.

3. Bake cookies 10 to 12 minutes, or until golden brown. Let cool 2 minutes on sheets, then remove to racks.

4. In a glass measuring cup, melt chocolate chips in a microwave or a pan of hot, not boiling, water. Stir sour cream and liqueur into melted chocolate. Dot centers of cookies with chocolate mixture. Let cool completely, then pack between layers of wax paper in a tightly covered container and store in refrigerator.

69   CARAMEL SURPRISES
Prep: 10 minutes   Bake: 8 to 10 minutes   Makes: 48

2   sticks (8 ounces) butter,
     softened
½   cup firmly packed dark
     brown sugar
1   teaspoon vanilla extract
1   teaspoon almond extract

2¼   cups cake flour
¼   teaspoon salt
⅓   cup finely ground almonds
12   caramel candies, cut into
     quarters
½   cup powdered sugar

1. Preheat oven to 375°F. In a medium bowl, beat butter and brown sugar with an electric mixer on medium speed until light and fluffy. Beat in vanilla and almond extract.

2. Add cake flour, salt, and almonds and mix until blended.

3. Shape dough into 1-inch balls. Press a piece of caramel into center of each ball and pinch dough to enclose. Place 1 inch apart on ungreased cookie sheets. Bake 8 to 10 minutes, or until edges just begin to turn golden brown. Remove to a wire rack to cool slightly, about 10 minutes. Roll in powdered sugar. Let cool completely.

70   BUTTER CHESTNUTS
Prep: 10 minutes   Bake: 12 to 15 minutes   Makes: about 42

1½ sticks (6 ounces) butter, softened
⅓ cup granulated sugar
1 teaspoon vanilla extract
1⅓ cups flour

1 cup ground hazelnuts or walnuts
3 tablespoons unsweetened cocoa powder
2 tablespoons powdered sugar

1. Preheat oven to 350°F. In a medium bowl, beat butter, granulated sugar, and vanilla with an electric mixer on medium speed until well blended. Beat in flour and nuts until dough is smooth, scraping side of bowl frequently with a rubber spatula.

2. Divide dough into 1¼-inch balls; flatten slightly. Arrange balls 2 inches apart on prepared baking sheets. Bake 12 to 15 minutes, or until lightly browned. Let cookies cool 2 minutes on sheets, then transfer to a wire rack set over a sheet of wax paper.

3. In a small bowl, combine cocoa powder and powdered sugar. Stir until well mixed. Sift cocoa mixture over warm cookies to coat tops completely. If necessary, place cocoa mixture that has fallen on wax paper back into sifter and sift onto cookies. Let cookies cool completely; store in a tightly covered container.

71   CHERRY SNOWDROPS
*Prep: 10 minutes   Chill: 1 hour   Bake: 10 to 12 minutes
Makes: about 36*

1 stick (4 ounces) plus 2 tablespoons butter, softened
½ cup granulated sugar
1 egg
1 teaspoon vanilla extract

½ teaspoon grated nutmeg
½ teaspoon salt
2¼ cups flour
½ cup dried sweet cherries, finely chopped
½ cup powdered sugar

1. In a medium bowl, beat butter and granulated sugar with an electric mixer on medium speed until light and fluffy. Beat in egg, vanilla, nutmeg, and salt until well blended.

2. Add flour and mix until blended. Stir in chopped cherries. Cover and refrigerate at least 1 hour, until firm.

3. Preheat oven to 350°F. Shape dough into 1-inch balls and place 2 inches apart on ungreased cookie sheets. Bake 10 to 12 minutes, until edges just begin to brown lightly.

4. Let stand 2 minutes on cookie sheets, then remove to a wire rack and let cool completely. Roll in powdered sugar before serving.

72   CHOCOLATE CRISPS
Prep: 5 minutes   Bake: 20 to 25 minutes   Makes: 24

2 sticks (8 ounces) butter,
    softened
⅔ cup superfine sugar
1¾ cups cake flour
½ cup unsweetened cocoa
    powder

½ teaspoon salt
2 teaspoons vanilla extract
¼ cup granulated sugar

1. Preheat oven to 325°F. In a medium bowl, beat butter and superfine sugar with an electric mixer on medium speed until light and fluffy. Add flour, cocoa, and salt and mix until blended.

2. Squeeze dough into a ball and divide in half. Press each half into an 8-inch disk about ½ inch thick on an ungreased cookie sheet. Crimp edges and prick all over with fork. Using a knife, cut each disk into 12 wedges. Sprinkle granulated sugar evenly over dough.

3. Bake 20 to 25 minutes, until set but not browned. Let cool in pan on a wire rack 5 minutes, then recut into wedges. Let cool completely on rack.

73   CHOCOLATE BRANDY BALLS
Prep: 10 minutes   Chill: 2 hours or overnight
Bake: 15 to 20 minutes   Makes: about 36

These brandy-infused cookies are an ideal ending for any holiday dinner.

1 stick (4 ounces) butter,
    softened
½ cup firmly packed dark
    brown sugar
¼ cup brandy
1 cup flour
¼ cup unsweetened cocoa
    powder

Pinch of salt
⅓ cup semisweet mini
    chocolate chips or finely
    chopped chocolate
1¼ cups finely chopped pecans
1 egg white, lightly beaten

1. In a medium bowl, beat butter and brown sugar with an electric mixer on medium speed until light and fluffy. Blend in brandy.

2. In a small bowl, stir together flour, cocoa, and salt until well mixed. Gradually beat into butter-sugar mixture until well blended. Stir in chocolate chips and ¼ cup pecans. Cover dough, which will be very sticky, with wax paper and refrigerate for 2 hours or overnight to firm up.

3. Preheat oven to 350°F. Using hands, shape about 2 teaspoons of dough at a time into 1-inch balls. Roll each ball in egg white, then in chopped nuts. Place ½ inch apart on greased cookie sheets.

4. Bake 15 to 20 minutes, until lightly crusted. Let stand 5 minutes, then remove to a wire rack and let cool completely.

74   CHOCOLATE SPRITZ COOKIES
Prep: 10 minutes   Bake: 10 to 12 minutes   Makes: about 36

1½ sticks (6 ounces) butter,
    softened
⅔ cup sugar
1 egg
2 (1-ounce) squares
    unsweetened chocolate,
    melted

1 teaspoon vanilla extract
2 cups flour
¼ teaspoon salt

1. Preheat oven to 350°F. In a medium bowl, beat butter, sugar, egg, chocolate, and vanilla with an electric mixer on medium speed until well blended.

2. Beat in flour and salt until dough is smooth, scraping down side of bowl frequently with a rubber spatula.

3. Spoon dough into a cookie press fitted with template of desired shape or a large pastry bag fitted with a large star or flower tip.

4. Press or pipe cookies 2 inches apart onto lightly greased cookie sheets. Bake 10 to 12 minutes, or until firm. Let cookies cool 2 minutes on sheets, then remove to wire racks and let cool completely. Store in a tightly covered container.

75   CHOCOLATE ALMOND SURPRISES
Prep: 20 minutes   Chill: 30 minutes   Bake: 10 minutes
Makes: about 48

2 sticks (8 ounces) butter,
    softened
1 cup granulated sugar
½ cup firmly packed dark
    brown sugar
2 eggs
1 teaspoon vanilla extract
1 teaspoon almond extract

3½ cups flour
1 teaspoon baking soda
½ teaspoon salt
8 ounces almond paste
½ cup semisweet chocolate
    chips
½ cup powdered sugar

1. In a medium bowl, beat together butter, granulated sugar, and brown sugar with an electric mixer on medium speed until light and fluffy. Add eggs, one at a time, beating well after each addition. Blend in vanilla and almond extract.

2. In a small bowl, stir together flour, baking soda, and salt until well mixed. Add to butter-sugar mixture and blend well. Cover and refrigerate dough 30 minutes, or until firm.

3. Preheat oven to 350°F. Using about ¼ teaspoon almond paste at a time, shape into 48 equal-size balls. Press 3 or 4 chocolate chips into almond paste. Wrap about 1 tablespoon chilled dough around each ball of filling, pinching to enclose completely.

4. Place about 2 inches apart on greased cookie sheets. Bake 10 minutes, or until lightly browned. Let stand 2 minutes on cookie sheets, then remove to a rack to cool. When cool, roll in powdered sugar.

---

76 CHOCOLATE RAVIOLI
Prep: 20 minutes   Chill: 30 minutes   Bake: 12 to 15 minutes
Makes: 24

Reminiscent of the pasta variety only in shape, these decadent morsels have a melt-in-your-mouth chocolate center.

1½ cups sugar	2¼ cups flour
1 stick (4 ounces) butter, softened	½ teaspoon baking powder
	¼ teaspoon salt
½ cup sour cream	4 ounces semisweet chocolate
1 egg	3 tablespoons ground almonds or hazelnuts
1½ teaspoons vanilla extract	

1. In a medium bowl, beat sugar and butter with an electric mixer on medium speed until well blended. Refrigerate ¼ cup sour cream, covered. Beat in remaining ¼ cup sour cream, egg, and vanilla until light and fluffy.

2. On low speed, beat in flour mixed with baking powder and salt until dough is smooth, scraping down side of bowl frequently with a rubber spatula. Divide dough in half; wrap in wax paper and refrigerate at least 30 minutes.

3. Just before baking, melt chocolate over hot, not boiling, water or in a microwave. Reserve 1 tablespoon. Stir reserved sour cream into remaining melted chocolate. Set aside.

4. Preheat oven to 350°F. Between pieces of wax paper, roll out each half of dough to make an 8½ × 12½-inch rectangle. Place one rectangle in freezer. Remove top sheet of wax paper from remaining sheet of dough. Drop chocolate mixture by heaping ½-teaspoon measures onto dough, spacing evenly, to make filling for 6 lengthwise rows of 4 ravioli. Remove dough from freezer; pull off one sheet of wax paper and place dough over chocolate on first sheet of dough. Allow dough to thaw and fall down over chocolate filling; remove top wax paper. With a fluted pastry wheel or a knife, trim edge of rectangle and cut between rows of chocolate filling to make 24 ravioli.

5. Place ravioli 2 inches apart on lightly greased cookie sheets. Bake 12 to 15 minutes, or until edges are golden brown. Let cookies cool 2 minutes on sheets, then remove to racks. Drizzle reserved chocolate over cookies; sprinkle ground nuts over chocolate. Let cool completely. Store between layers of wax paper in a tightly covered container.

77   CHOCOLATE CRACKLE KISSES
Prep: 10 minutes   Cook: 2 to 3 minutes   Bake: 12 to 15 minutes
Makes: about 48

The kids will enjoy helping to make these almost as much as eating them.

4 tablespoons butter	1½ cups flour
3 (1-ounce) squares unsweetened chocolate	2 teaspoons baking powder
1 cup granulated sugar	¼ teaspoon salt
2 eggs	⅓ cup powdered sugar
1 teaspoon vanilla extract	48 chocolate kisses

1. Preheat oven to 350°F. In a heatproof bowl in a microwave oven on High power or in a double boiler over hot water, melt butter and chocolate, 2 to 3 minutes. Stir until smooth and well blended.

2. In a medium bowl, with an electric mixer on medium speed, beat butter and chocolate with sugar until blended. Beat in eggs and vanilla.

3. Add flour mixed with baking powder and salt and beat on low speed until blended.

4. Form dough into 1-inch balls, roll in powdered sugar, and place 2 inches apart on ungreased cookie sheets.

5. Bake 12 to 15 minutes, or until edges are set. Remove from oven and immediately press a chocolate kiss pointed side up into center of each cookie. Let stand 2 minutes, then remove to a rack and let cool completely.

78   CHOCOLATE PEANUT BUTTER COOKIES
Prep: 10 minutes   Chill: 30 minutes   Bake: 10 to 12 minutes
Makes: about 48

Chocolate makes these peanut butter cookies even more irresistible, especially to kids.

1 stick (4 ounces) butter, softened	2 (1-ounce) squares unsweetened chocolate, melted
½ cup creamy peanut butter	
¾ cup granulated sugar	1⅓ cups flour
6 tablespoons firmly packed dark brown sugar	½ teaspoon baking powder
	½ teaspoon baking soda
1 egg	½ teaspoon salt
1 teaspoon vanilla extract	

1. In a medium bowl, beat butter and peanut butter with an electric mixer on medium speed until creamy. Add granulated sugar and brown sugar and beat until blended. Beat in egg, vanilla, and melted chocolate until well blended.

2. Add flour mixed with baking powder, baking soda, and salt and beat until well blended. Cover and refrigerate until firm, about 30 minutes.

3. Preheat oven to 350°F. Shape dough into 1-inch balls and place 1 inch apart on greased cookie sheets. Flatten with a fork. Bake 10 to 12 minutes, or until cookies are set. Let cool on sheets 2 minutes, then remove to a rack and let cool completely.

---

79 CHOCOLATE PEPPERMINT DROPS

Prep: 10 minutes   Chill: 1 hour   Bake: 8 to 10 minutes
Makes: about 48

2 sticks (8 ounces) butter, softened
¾ cup sugar
1 egg
2 (1-ounce) squares unsweetened chocolate, melted
1 teaspoon vanilla extract

½ teaspoon peppermint extract
2½ cups flour
1 teaspoon baking powder
¼ teaspoon salt
About ¼ cup mint chocolate chips

1. In a medium bowl, beat butter and sugar with an electric mixer on medium speed until light and fluffy. Beat in egg, chocolate, vanilla, and peppermint extract.

2. Add flour mixed with baking powder and salt and beat until blended. Cover and refrigerate at least 1 hour, until firm.

3. Preheat oven to 375°F. Shape dough into 1-inch balls and place 1 inch apart on ungreased cookie sheets. Place one mint chocolate chip in the center of each ball and press gently to flatten.

4. Bake 8 to 10 minutes, or until edges just begin to brown. Let stand 2 minutes, then remove to a rack and let cool completely.

80   CHOCOLATE WAFERS

Prep: 10 minutes   Chill: 2 hours   Bake: 10 to 12 minutes
Makes: about 36

1½ sticks (6 ounces) butter,
    softened
¾ cup sugar
1 egg
1 teaspoon vanilla extract

1¾ cups flour
¼ cup unsweetened cocoa
    powder
¼ teaspoon salt

1. In a large bowl, beat butter and sugar with an electric mixer on medium speed until well blended. Beat in egg and vanilla until light and fluffy.

2. On low speed, beat in flour, cocoa, and salt until dough is smooth, scraping down side of bowl frequently with a rubber spatula. Wrap dough in wax paper and refrigerate 2 to 3 hours, until firm.

3. Preheat oven to 350°F. Divide dough into 1-inch balls. With floured hands, flatten dough balls into 2-inch rounds and place 2 inches apart on lightly greased cookie sheets.

4. Bake 10 to 12 minutes, or until wafers are firm. Let cool 2 minutes on sheets, then remove to wire racks and let cool completely.

81   COCOA KRINKLES

Prep: 10 minutes   Chill: 2 hours   Bake: 15 to 17 minutes
Makes: about 48

2⅓ cups flour
2 teaspoons baking powder
½ teaspoon salt
2 cups granulated sugar
¾ cup vegetable oil

¾ cup unsweetened cocoa
    powder
4 eggs
2 teaspoons vanilla extract
¼ cup powdered sugar
¼ teaspoon cinnamon

1. In a small bowl, stir together flour, baking powder, and salt until well mixed. In a large bowl, combine granulated sugar and oil. Mix in cocoa, then beat in eggs and vanilla. Add flour mixture and blend well. Wrap dough in wax paper and refrigerate 2 hours or overnight to firm up.

2. Preheat oven to 350°F. In a small bowl, mix powdered sugar and cinnamon. Using your hands, shape dough into 1-inch balls, roll in cinnamon sugar, then place 2 inches apart on greased cookie sheets.

3. Bake 15 to 17 minutes, or until cooked through. Let stand 5 minutes, remove to a wire rack, and let cool completely.

82 COCONUT KRINKLES
Prep: 10 minutes   Chill: 1 hour   Bake: 12 to 15 minutes
Makes: about 24

1 stick (4 ounces) butter, softened
½ cup powdered sugar
1 teaspoon vanilla extract
1 teaspoon almond extract

¾ cup plus 2 tablespoons cake flour
½ teaspoon salt
⅓ cup finely ground almonds
½ cup flaked coconut

1. In a medium bowl, beat butter and powdered sugar with an electric mixer on medium speed until light and fluffy. Beat in vanilla and almond extract until well blended.

2. Add cake flour, salt, and almonds and beat until blended. Stir in coconut and mix well. Tightly wrap in wax paper and refrigerate at least 1 hour, or until firm.

3. Preheat oven to 350°F. Shape dough into 1-inch balls and place 1 inch apart on ungreased cookie sheets. Bake 12 to 15 minutes, until edges begin to color. Let cookies cool on sheets 2 minutes, then remove to a rack and let cool completely.

83 COCONUT TEA CAKES
Prep: 10 minutes   Bake: 8 to 9 minutes   Makes: about 48

2 sticks (8 ounces) butter, softened
1 cup powdered sugar
1 teaspoon almond extract
1 teaspoon vanilla extract
2¼ cups cake flour

¼ teaspoon salt
⅓ cup finely ground almonds
1 tablespoon grated lemon zest
¾ cup flaked coconut, toasted

1. Preheat oven to 375°F. In a medium bowl, beat butter and ½ cup powdered sugar with an electric mixer on medium speed until light and fluffy. Beat in almond extract and vanilla.

2. Add cake flour, salt, almonds, and lemon zest and mix until blended. Stir in coconut.

3. Shape dough into 1-inch balls and place 1 inch apart on ungreased cookie sheets. Bake 8 to 9 minutes, or until edges just begin to turn golden brown. Remove to a wire rack to cool slightly, about 10 minutes. Roll in remaining ½ cup powdered sugar. Let cool completely.

84   CORN RUSKS

Prep: 15 minutes   Rise: 50 to 60 minutes   Bake: 40 to 42 minutes
Stand: 45 minutes   Makes: about 60

These crisp double-baked cookies are a good accompaniment to port, sherry, or Madeira.

1 (¼-ounce) envelope active dry yeast	¼ cup vegetable oil
1¼ cups lukewarm water (105° to 115°)	1 egg
½ cup sugar	½ teaspoon salt
	1½ cups cornmeal
	2½ to 3 cups flour

1. In a large bowl, combine yeast and ½ cup warm water. Set aside 5 minutes for yeast to soften. Beat in remaining warm water, sugar, oil, egg, and salt.

2. Add cornmeal and 2½ cups flour. Beat with an electric mixer on medium speed, scraping down side of bowl frequently with a rubber spatula, until well blended. Knead dough in bowl with your hands, adding more flour if necessary, until a smooth, soft dough forms, about 5 minutes.

3. Divide dough into quarters. Shape each quarter into a 9 × 2-inch log and set logs 3 inches apart on a greased cookie sheet. Allow to rise in a warm, draftfree place, lightly covered with a kitchen towel, 50 to 60 minutes, or until doubled in size. Meanwhile, preheat oven to 350°F.

4. Bake raised logs 30 minutes, or until golden brown. Remove from oven; leave oven on. Let logs stand on a wire rack 10 to 15 minutes, or until cool enough to handle.

5. With a serrated knife, cut each log into 15 slices. Place slices flat on ungreased cookie sheets, return to oven, and bake 5 minutes. Turn slices over and bake 5 to 7 minutes longer, or until golden on both sides. Turn off oven and leave rusks without opening door until oven is cool, about 45 minutes. Remove rusks to racks and let cool completely. Store in a tightly covered container.

85   GINGER AND SPICE COOKIES

Prep: 10 minutes   Chill: 1 hour   Bake: 10 to 12 minutes
Makes: about 36

2 cups flour	1¼ cups sugar
1 teaspoon baking soda	¾ cup solid vegetable shortening
½ teaspoon salt	
1 teaspoon cinnamon	¼ cup light molasses
1 teaspoon ground ginger	1 egg
½ teaspoon ground allspice	

1. In a small bowl, stir together flour, baking soda, salt, cinnamon, ginger, and allspice.

2. In a medium bowl, beat sugar and shortening with an electric mixer on medium speed until light and fluffy. Beat in molasses and egg.

3. Add flour mixture to sugar mixture and beat until well blended. Cover and refrigerate dough at least 1 hour, until firm.

4. Preheat oven to 350°F. Roll dough into 1-inch balls and place 2 inches apart on ungreased cookie sheets. Flatten slightly, using the tines of a fork. Bake 10 to 12 minutes, just until golden brown. Let stand 2 minutes on cookie sheet, then remove to a wire rack and let cool completely.

---

86 GRAHAM DROPS
Prep: 15 minutes   Bake: 6 to 8 minutes   Makes: 36

This is an old-fashioned graham cracker recipe turned into a bite-size treat. Whole wheat flour is sometimes called graham flour.

1 cup all-purpose flour	2 tablespoons solid vegetable
½ cup whole wheat flour	shortening
2 tablespoons firmly packed	3 tablespoons butter
dark brown sugar	1 tablespoon honey
½ teaspoon baking soda	1 tablespoon molasses
¼ teaspoon salt	1 teaspoon vanilla extract
½ teaspoon cinnamon	About ¼ cup raspberry jam

1. In a medium bowl, combine flour, whole wheat flour, brown sugar, baking soda, salt, and cinnamon. Using a pastry cutter, 2 knives, or your fingers, cut in shortening and butter until crumbly.

2. In a small bowl, combine honey, molasses, vanilla, and 2 tablespoons water. Stir until well mixed. Gradually stir into dry ingredients, tossing with a fork until dough begins to cling together. Press dough together.

3. Shape dough into 1-inch balls and place 1 inch apart on ungreased cookie sheets. Make a deep thumbprint in the centers and fill each with a scant ½ teaspoon jam.

4. Bake 6 to 8 minutes, or until edges just begin to turn golden brown. Let stand 2 minutes, then remove to a wire rack and let cool completely.

87   HAZELNUT BALLS

Prep: 10 minutes   Chill: 1 hour   Bake: 25 to 30 minutes
Makes: about 36

These melt-in-your-mouth balls are sure to become a family favorite.

1   cup toasted hazelnuts
1   cup cake flour
½   cup plus ¼ cup powdered
    sugar

1   stick (4 ounces) butter,
    softened
¼   cup superfine sugar
1   teaspoon vanilla extract

1. In a food processor, blend hazelnuts, flour, and ¼ cup powdered sugar until hazelnuts are finely ground.

2. In a medium bowl, beat butter and superfine sugar with an electric mixer on medium speed until light and fluffy. Beat in vanilla.

3. Add nut mixture to sugar mixture and beat until blended. Cover and refrigerate at least 1 hour, until firm.

4. Preheat oven to 300°F. Shape dough into ¾-inch balls and place 1 inch apart on greased cookie sheets. Bake 25 to 30 minutes, or until cookies are set and look faintly golden.

5. Remove cookies to a wire rack and let cool slightly, about 5 minutes. Roll in ½ cup powdered sugar. Let cookies cool completely, then roll again in powdered sugar.

88   HAZELNUT MELTAWAYS

Prep: 15 minutes   Chill: 1 hour   Bake: 12 to 15 minutes
Makes: about 36

2   sticks (8 ounces) unsalted
    butter, softened
¾   cup plus ½ cup powdered
    sugar
2   teaspoons vanilla extract

Pinch of salt
2   cups flour
1   cup finely chopped toasted
    hazelnuts

1. In a medium bowl, beat butter and ¾ cup powdered sugar with an electric mixer on medium speed until light and fluffy. Beat in vanilla and salt until well blended.

2. Add flour to sugar mixture and blend well. Stir in hazelnuts. Cover and refrigerate at least 1 hour, until firm.

3. Preheat oven to 350°F. Shape 2 teaspoonfuls of dough at a time into crescents about 3 inches long and place 2 inches apart on ungreased cookie sheets.

4. Bake 12 to 15 minutes, or until edges of cookies just begin to brown lightly. Let cool 5 minutes on cookie sheets, then roll in remaining ½ cup powdered sugar, transfer to a wire rack, and let cool completely.

89 HAZELNUT AMBROSIA WEDDING CAKES
Prep: 10 minutes   Chill: 1 hour   Bake: 15 to 20 minutes
Makes: about 42

2 sticks (8 ounces) butter,
  softened
¾ cup plus ½ cup powdered
  sugar
1 teaspoon vanilla extract

2 cups flour
¾ cup finely chopped toasted
  hazelnuts
¼ cup flaked coconut
1 teaspoon grated orange zest

1. In a medium bowl, beat butter and ¾ cup powdered sugar with an electric mixer on medium speed until light and fluffy. Beat in vanilla.

2. Add flour and mix until blended. Stir in hazelnuts, coconut, and orange zest. Cover and refrigerate at least 1 hour, until firm.

3. Preheat oven to 325°F. Shape dough into ½-inch balls and place 1 inch apart on ungreased cookie sheets. Bake 15 to 20 minutes, or until edges just begin to turn golden brown. Remove to a wire rack and let cool slightly, about 10 minutes. Roll in ½ cup powdered sugar. Let cool completely.

90 HAZELNUT DELIGHTS
Prep: 20 minutes   Chill: 10 to 15 minutes   Bake: 30 minutes
Makes: 64

2 cups flour
2 sticks (8 ounces) butter,
  softened
6 ounces cream cheese,
  softened
½ teaspoon salt
1 cup firmly packed dark
  brown sugar

¾ cup finely chopped
  hazelnuts
2 eggs, lightly beaten
1 tablespoon melted butter
1 teaspoon vanilla extract
  Pinch of salt
64 whole hazelnuts (about
  ½ cup), for garnish

1. In a medium bowl, beat flour, butter, cream cheese, and salt with an electric mixer on medium speed until well blended. Scoop up dough into level measuring tablespoons and roll into 16 equal-sized balls about 1¼ inches in diameter. Place 2 inches apart on an ungreased cookie sheet. Using a finger dipped in flour, make a deep indentation in each ball to form a bowl shape. Place into the freezer for 10 to 15 minutes to firm up dough.

2. Preheat oven to 350°F. In a small bowl, stir together brown sugar, hazelnuts, eggs, butter, vanilla, and salt. Remove dough from freezer and fill each indentation with about 1 teaspoon of sugar-nut mixture. Top each with a hazelnut.

3. Bake for 30 minutes, or until lightly browned. Let cool completely on wire racks.

91   HIDDEN TREASURES

Prep: 10 minutes   Bake: 8 to 10 minutes   Makes: about 48

One bite reveals the chocolate hidden inside these butter balls.

1 cup firmly packed dark
   brown sugar
¾ cup powdered sugar
2 sticks (8 ounces) butter,
   softened
2 eggs

1 teaspoon vanilla extract
3 cups cake flour
1 teaspoon baking powder
½ teaspoon salt
About ¾ cup chocolate chips

1. Preheat oven to 375°F. In a medium bowl, beat brown sugar, powdered sugar, and butter with an electric mixer on medium speed until light and fluffy. Beat in eggs and vanilla.

2. Add cake flour mixed with baking powder and salt. Stir until blended. Shape about a tablespoon of dough around a few chocolate chips. Place dough balls 2 inches apart on ungreased cookie sheets.

3. Bake 8 to 10 minutes, or until edges just begin to turn golden brown. Let stand 2 minutes before removing to a rack to cool completely.

---

92   LEMON PRETZELS

Prep: 15 minutes   Chill: 1 hour   Bake: 8 to 10 minutes   Makes: 32

These lemony cookies are as tasty as they are attractive.

1 stick (4 ounces) butter,
   softened
½ cup plus ⅓ cup sugar
1 egg
1 teaspoon vanilla extract

½ teaspoon lemon extract
2½ teaspoons grated lemon zest
1¼ cups flour
½ teaspoon baking powder
¼ teaspoon salt

1. In a medium bowl, beat butter and ½ cup sugar with an electric mixer on medium speed until light and fluffy. Beat in egg, vanilla, lemon extract, and 2 teaspoons lemon zest.

2. Mix together flour, baking powder, and salt. Add to sugar mixture and beat until blended. Cover and refrigerate at least 1 hour, until firm.

3. Preheat oven to 375°F. In a wide, shallow bowl, stir together remaining ⅓ cup sugar and ½ teaspoon lemon zest. Divide one fourth of dough into 8 pieces. Roll each piece into a 6-inch-long strip, twist strip into a pretzel (see Note), or tie in a knot. Dip top of pretzels in lemon sugar and place 1 inch apart on ungreased cookie sheet. Repeat with remaining dough.

4. Bake 8 to 10 minutes, or until edges just begin to turn golden brown. Transfer to a rack and let cool.

NOTE: *To form pretzels, place dough rope on a flat work surface in a U shape, like a horseshoe with ends toward you. Lift ends, twist, and turn back toward bend of U. Spread ends apart and press onto dough about ¼ inch on either side of center of bend.*

93 LEMON SPRITZ COOKIES
Prep: 15 minutes   Bake: 10 to 12 minutes   Makes: about 40

1½ sticks (6 ounces) butter,
    softened
1 cup powdered sugar
3 tablespoons lemon juice

1 teaspoon finely grated
    lemon zest
2¼ cups flour
¼ teaspoon salt

1. Preheat oven to 350°F. In a medium bowl, beat butter, powdered sugar, lemon juice, and lemon zest with an electric mixer on medium speed until well blended.

2. Beat in flour and salt until dough is smooth, scraping down side of bowl frequently with a rubber spatula.

3. Spoon dough into a cookie press fitted with template of desired shape or a large pastry bag fitted with a large star or flower tip. Press or pipe cookies 2 inches apart onto lightly greased cookie sheets.

4. Bake 10 to 12 minutes, or until golden brown. Let cookies cool 2 minutes on sheets, then remove to racks and let cool completely. Store in a tightly covered container.

---

94 MINT CHOCOLATE LOGS
Prep: 15 minutes   Chill: 1 hour   Bake: 8 to 10 minutes   Makes: 48

1 stick (4 ounces) butter,
    softened
4 ounces cream cheese,
    softened
¾ cup sugar
1 egg yolk
1 (1-ounce) square
    unsweetened chocolate,
    melted

½ teaspoon vanilla extract
½ teaspoon peppermint extract
1½ cups flour
¼ cup finely ground almonds
½ teaspoon baking powder
¼ teaspoon salt
½ cup mint chocolate chips,
    melted

1. In a medium bowl, beat butter, cream cheese, and sugar with an electric mixer on medium speed until light and fluffy. Beat in egg yolk, melted chocolate, vanilla, and peppermint extract.

2. Add flour mixed with almonds, baking powder, and salt and beat until blended. Cover and refrigerate at least 1 hour, until firm.

3. Preheat oven to 375°F. Divide one fourth of dough into 12 pieces. Roll each piece into 2½-inch-long strip and place the strips 1 inch apart on ungreased cookie sheets. Repeat with remaining dough.

4. Bake 8 to 10 minutes, or until edges are set. Let cookies cool on sheets 2 minutes, then remove to a rack and let cool completely. Using a knife or a metal spatula, spread melted chocolate on one end of each log.

95   MOCHA-NUT MELTAWAYS

Prep: 10 minutes   Chill: 1 hour   Bake: 15 to 18 minutes
Makes: about 36

2 sticks (8 ounces) unsalted
   butter, softened
6 tablespoons granulated
   sugar
1 teaspoon instant coffee
   powder
1 teaspoon unsweetened
   cocoa powder

1 teaspoon almond extract
½ teaspoon cinnamon
¼ teaspoon salt
2 cups flour
1 cup finely chopped almonds
½ cup powdered sugar

1. In a medium bowl, beat butter and granulated sugar with an electric mixer on medium speed until light and fluffy. Beat in coffee powder, cocoa, almond extract, cinnamon, and salt until well blended.

2. Add flour and mix until blended. Stir in almonds. Cover and refrigerate at least 1 hour, until firm.

3. Preheat oven to 350°F. Shape dough into 1-inch balls and place 2 inches apart on ungreased cookie sheets. Bake 15 to 18 minutes, or until edges just begin to brown lightly. Let cool 5 minutes on cookie sheet, roll in powdered sugar, remove to a wire rack, and let cool completely. Then roll again in powdered sugar.

96   MOLASSES SPICE KISSES

Prep: 15 minutes   Chill: 1 hour   Bake: 6 to 8 minutes   Makes: 48

1 stick (4 ounces) butter,
   softened
¾ cup firmly packed dark
   brown sugar
1 egg yolk
1 tablespoon dark molasses
½ teaspoon vanilla extract
1½ cups flour

½ teaspoon baking soda
¼ teaspoon salt
1 teaspoon cinnamon
1 teaspoon ground ginger
½ teaspoon grated nutmeg
½ teaspoon ground allspice
½ cup powdered sugar

1. In a medium bowl, beat butter and brown sugar with an electric mixer on medium speed until light and fluffy. Beat in egg yolk, molasses, and vanilla.

2. Add flour mixed with baking soda, salt, cinnamon, ginger, nutmeg, and allspice and beat until blended. Cover and refrigerate at least 1 hour, or until firm.

3. Preheat oven to 400°F. Divide one fourth of dough into 12 pieces. Roll each piece into a 1-inch ball and place balls 1 inch apart on ungreased cookie sheets. Repeat with remaining dough.

4. Bake 6 to 8 minutes, or until cooked through. Let cookies cool on sheets 2 minutes, then remove to a rack and let cool completely. Sprinkle powdered sugar over tops of cookies.

97   MACADAMIA MADNESS
Prep: 20 minutes   Chill: 10 to 15 minutes   Bake: 30 minutes
Makes: about 64

- 2 cups flour
- 2 sticks (8 ounces) butter, softened
- 6 ounces cream cheese, softened
- ½ teaspoon salt
- ½ cup firmly packed dark brown sugar
- ½ cup granulated sugar
- ½ cup finely chopped toasted almonds
- ¼ cup chopped macadamia nuts
- 2 eggs, lightly beaten
- 1 tablespoon melted butter
- 1 teaspoon grated lemon zest
- 1 teaspoon vanilla extract
- ¼ teaspoon lemon extract
- Pinch of salt
- 64 whole macadamia nuts (about ⅔ cup)

1. In a medium bowl, beat flour, butter, cream cheese, and salt with an electric mixer on medium speed until well blended. Scoop up level measuring tablespoons of dough and roll into 1¼-inch balls. Place on ungreased cookie sheets. Using a finger dipped in flour, make a deep indentation in each ball to form a bowl shape. Place in the freezer for 10 to 15 minutes to firm up dough.

2. Preheat oven to 350°F. In a small bowl, stir together brown sugar, granulated sugar, almonds, chopped macadamia nuts, eggs, butter, lemon zest, vanilla, lemon extract, and salt. Remove cookie sheets from freezer and fill each indentation with about 1 teaspoon of sugar-nut mixture. Top each with a macadamia nut.

3. Bake for 30 minutes, or until lightly browned. Let cool completely on wire racks.

98   SESAME BREAKFAST RINGS
Prep: 20 minutes   Bake: 12 to 15 minutes   Makes: 42

These not-too-sweet cookies make the perfect breakfast compromise for those who never have time for breakfast and just grab a quick coffee.

1 cup sugar	¼ teaspoon salt
1 stick (4 ounces) butter, softened	½ cup milk
	½ teaspoon vanilla extract
2 whole eggs	1 egg yolk
5 cups flour	3 tablespoons sesame seeds
1 teaspoon baking powder	

1. Preheat oven to 350°F. In a large bowl, beat sugar and butter with an electric mixer on medium speed until well blended. Beat in 2 whole eggs until light and fluffy.

2. On low speed, beat in flour mixed with baking powder and salt, alternately with milk and vanilla, until dough is smooth, scraping down side of bowl frequently with a rubber spatula.

3. Divide dough into 42 pieces. With palms of hands, roll each piece of dough into a 7-inch rope. In a small bowl, beat egg yolk with a few drops of water. Spread sesame seeds on a saucer. Shape each rope into a ring and pinch edges together to seal. Brush tops with egg yolk mixture, dip into sesame seeds, and place, seeded-side up, on lightly greased cookie sheets.

4. Bake 12 to 15 minutes, or until firm and very lightly browned. Remove rings to a rack and let cool completely. Store in a tightly covered container.

99   ORANGE CANDY DROPS
Prep: 15 minutes   Chill: 1 hour   Bake: 8 to 10 minutes   Makes: 32

These orange cookies are so sweet it's almost like eating candy.

1 stick (4 ounces) butter, softened	2 teaspoons grated orange zest
	1¼ cups flour
1 cup granulated sugar	½ teaspoon baking powder
1 egg	¼ teaspoon salt
1 teaspoon vanilla extract	½ cup powdered sugar
½ teaspoon orange extract	

1. Preheat oven to 375°F. In a medium bowl, beat butter and granulated sugar with an electric mixer on medium speed until light and fluffy. Beat in egg, vanilla, orange extract, and orange zest.

2. Add flour mixed with baking powder and salt and beat until blended. Divide one fourth of dough into 8 pieces. Roll each piece into a ball and place balls 1 inch apart on an ungreased cookie sheet. Repeat with remaining dough.

3. Bake 8 to 10 minutes, or until edges just begin to turn golden brown. Dip warm cookies into powdered sugar. Let cool completely on a rack.

100   RASPBERRY-COCONUT COOKIES
Prep: 10 minutes   Chill: 1 hour   Bake: 8 to 10 minutes
Makes: about 30

1 stick (4 ounces) butter,
  softened
½ cup powdered sugar
1 teaspoon vanilla extract
1 teaspoon almond extract

1 cup plus 2 tablespoons cake
  flour
½ cup flaked coconut
⅓ cup finely ground almonds
¼ cup raspberry jam

1. In a medium bowl, beat butter and powdered sugar with an electric mixer on medium speed until light and fluffy. Beat in vanilla and almond extract until well blended.

2. Add cake flour, coconut, and almonds and beat until blended. Tightly wrap in wax paper and refrigerate at least 1 hour, or until firm.

3. Preheat oven to 350°F. Shape dough into 1-inch balls and place 1 inch apart on ungreased cookie sheets. Bake 8 to 10 minutes, until bottoms begin to color.

4. Remove from oven and carefully make a deep indentation with a teaspoon in center of each cookie. Fill with a scant ½ teaspoon jam. Let cookies cool on sheets 2 minutes, then remove to rack to cool completely.

101   PEANUT SPICE COOKIES
Prep: 15 minutes   Bake: 12 to 15 minutes   Makes: about 48

1¼ cups finely chopped peanuts
1¼ cups sugar
2½ cups flour
2 teaspoons baking soda
1 teaspoon cinnamon
½ teaspoon ground ginger
½ teaspoon grated nutmeg

¼ teaspoon ground allspice
¼ teaspoon salt
1½ sticks (6 ounces) butter,
  softened
1 egg
⅓ cup dark molasses

1. Preheat oven to 350°F. Toss ½ cup peanuts with ¼ cup sugar. Set aside.

2. In a small bowl, stir together flour, baking soda, cinnamon, ginger, nutmeg, allspice, and salt.

3. In a large bowl, beat butter and remaining 1 cup sugar with an electric mixer on medium speed until creamy. Mix in remaining ¾ cup peanuts. Beat in egg, then molasses until well blended. Add flour mixture to butter-sugar mixture and beat until thoroughly combined.

4. Form dough into 1-inch balls, roll each in reserved peanut-sugar mixture, and place 2 inches apart on greased cookie sheets. Bake 12 to 15 minutes, until set around the edges. Let stand 3 minutes, then remove to a wire rack and let cool completely.

102 SESAME CHOCOLATE COOKIES
Prep: 10 minutes   Chill: 1 hour   Bake: 10 to 12 minutes
Makes: about 42

1 stick (4 ounces) butter,
  softened
½ cup sugar
2 tablespoons molasses
1 egg
2 (1-ounce) squares
  unsweetened chocolate,
  melted

¼ cup milk, at room
  temperature
2 cups flour
1 teaspoon baking powder
½ teaspoon salt
½ teaspoon ground ginger
¾ cup sesame seeds

1. In a medium bowl, beat butter and sugar with an electric mixer on medium speed until blended. Beat in molasses and egg until well blended. Blend in melted chocolate and then milk.

2. Add flour mixed with baking powder, salt, and ginger and beat on low speed until well blended. Cover dough and refrigerate until firm, about 1 hour.

3. Preheat oven to 375°F. Shape dough into 1-inch balls, roll in sesame seeds, and place 1 inch apart on greased cookie sheets. Flatten gently with bottom of a glass.

4. Bake 10 to 12 minutes, until cookies are set. Let cookies cool on sheet 2 minutes, then remove to a rack and let cool completely.

103 VANILLA SPRITZ COOKIES
Prep: 15 minutes   Bake: 10 to 12 minutes   Makes: about 36

1½ sticks (6 ounces) butter,
  softened
⅓ cup sugar
2 egg yolks

2 teaspoons vanilla extract
2 cups cake flour
¼ teaspoon salt

1. Preheat oven to 350°F. In a medium bowl, beat butter, sugar, egg yolks, and vanilla with an electric mixer on medium speed until well blended.

2. Add cake flour and salt and beat on low speed until dough is smooth, scraping down side of bowl frequently with a rubber spatula.

3. Spoon dough into a cookie press fitted with template of desired shape or a large pastry bag fitted with a large star or flower tip. Press or pipe cookies 2 inches apart onto lightly greased cookie sheets.

4. Bake 10 to 12 minutes, or until golden brown. Let cookies cool 2 minutes on sheets, then remove to racks and let cool completely. Store in a tightly covered container.

104 SURPRISE SHORTBREAD
Prep: 10 minutes   Bake: 10 to 15 minutes   Makes: 30

2 sticks (8 ounces) butter, softened	¼ teaspoon almond extract
½ cup sugar	2 cups flour
½ teaspoon vanilla extract	¼ teaspoon salt
	30 unblanched almonds

1. Preheat oven to 325°F. In a medium bowl, beat butter and sugar with an electric mixer on medium speed until light and fluffy. Beat in vanilla and almond extract.

2. Add flour and salt and mix until blended. Shape dough into 1-inch balls and insert an almond, leaving about one third of nut exposed. Place 1 inch apart on ungreased cookie sheets.

3. Bake 10 to 15 minutes, until cookies are pale golden, not brown. Let stand 2 minutes, then remove to a rack and let cool completely.

105 SPICY SPRITZ COOKIES
Prep: 15 minutes   Bake: 10 minutes   Makes: about 40

1½ sticks (6 ounces) butter, softened	1 teaspoon cinnamon
½ cup sugar	½ teaspoon ground ginger
1 egg	¼ teaspoon grated nutmeg
1 teaspoon vanilla extract	¼ teaspoon ground allspice
1¾ cups flour	¼ teaspoon salt

1. Preheat oven to 350°F. In a medium bowl, beat butter, sugar, egg, and vanilla with an electric mixer on medium speed until well blended.

2. Beat in flour mixed with cinnamon, ginger, nutmeg, allspice, and salt until dough is smooth, scraping down side of bowl frequently with a rubber spatula.

3. Spoon dough into a cookie press fitted with template of desired shape or a large pastry bag fitted with a large star or flower tip. Press or pipe cookies 2 inches apart onto lightly greased cookie sheets.

4. Bake 10 minutes, or until golden brown. Let cookies cool 2 minutes on sheets, then remove to racks and let cool completely. Store in a tightly covered container.

106 WHEAT 'N' HONEY PEANUT BUTTER COOKIES

Prep: 10 minutes   Bake: 12 to 15 minutes   Makes: about 42

1 cup whole wheat flour
¼ cup plus 2 tablespoons all-purpose flour
1 teaspoon baking powder
¼ teaspoon salt
1 stick (4 ounces) butter, softened

¼ cup plus 2 tablespoons crunchy peanut butter
½ cup firmly packed dark brown sugar
3 tablespoons honey
1 egg
1 teaspoon vanilla extract

1. In a small bowl, combine whole wheat flour, all-purpose flour, baking powder, and salt. Stir to blend.

2. In a medium bowl, beat butter and peanut butter with an electric mixer on medium speed until blended. Add brown sugar and honey and beat until light and fluffy. Beat in egg and vanilla.

3. Add flour to sugar mixture and stir until blended. If dough is too sticky to handle, cover and refrigerate about 15 minutes to chill.

4. Preheat oven to 350°F. Shape dough into 1-inch balls and place 2 inches apart on ungreased cookie sheets. Using a floured fork, flatten each cookie. Bake 12 to 15 minutes, or until edges just begin to turn golden brown. Remove to rack to cool completely.

Chapter 4

Ready and Waiting

One of the most convenient kinds of cookies to make is icebox, or refrigerator, cookies. Invented years ago by cooks who were just as busy as we are, refrigerator cookies can be made ahead, wrapped, and tucked away in the refrigerator to be baked at a more convenient time. Refrigerator cookie dough is best if used within 3 to 4 days when stored at refrigerator temperatures, but it can be kept in the freezer for up to 6 months. You may want to double the recipes in this chapter and put a roll of dough in the freezer for last-minute baking when needed.

Refrigerator cookies can be varied by changing the diameter of the rolls and by slicing them at different thicknesses. You can make very tiny rolls and bake up handfuls of little treats like our Butterscotch Pennies or make the rolls extra wide and cut them in quarters to make small fans to top a scoop of ice cream.

The doughs used for rolled cookies and refrigerator cookies are very much alike in proportions. If you want to make one of our rolled cookies but don't have the time, or the room, to roll and cut out shapes, you can make the dough, form it into rolls, refrigerate, and slice them instead.

One of the most welcoming aromas your home can have is that of cookies baking. If you have a roll of refrigerator cookies in your freezer, no matter how busy you are you can slice and bake a cookie welcome for unexpected guests, family members returning from a trip, or the children coming home from school.

107 APPLE BUTTER COOKIES

Prep: 10 minutes   Chill: 1 hour   Bake: 8 to 10 minutes
Makes: about 48

6 tablespoons butter, softened
6 tablespoons apple butter
½ cup plus ⅓ cup powdered
   sugar
1 teaspoon vanilla extract

1 cup plus 2 tablespoons flour
¼ teaspoon salt
2 to 3 teaspoons apple juice
   or apple brandy

1. In a medium bowl, beat butter, apple butter, and ½ cup powdered sugar with an electric mixer on medium speed until light and fluffy. Beat in vanilla until well blended.

2. Add flour and salt and beat until blended. Shape dough into 2 logs about 8 inches long. Wrap tightly in wax paper and refrigerate at least 1 hour, until firm.

3. Preheat oven to 400°F. Cut logs into ⅜-inch-thick slices and place 2 inches apart on ungreased cookie sheets. Bake 8 to 10 minutes, until bottoms begin to color. Let cookies cool on sheets 2 minutes, then remove to a rack and let cool completely.

4. In a small bowl, stir together remaining ⅓ cup powdered sugar and enough apple juice or brandy to make an icing of spreading consistency. Spread on completely cooled cookies.

108 BUTTERSCOTCH PENNIES

Prep: 10 minutes   Chill: 3 hours   Bake: 8 to 10 minutes per batch
Makes: about 160

You can eat these delicious little bites by the handful.

¾ cup packed brown sugar
1½ sticks (6 ounces) butter,
   softened
1 teaspoon vanilla extract

1¾ cups flour
½ teaspoon baking powder
¼ teaspoon salt

1. In a large bowl, beat brown sugar, butter, and vanilla with an electric mixer on medium speed until well blended. Beat in flour mixed with baking powder and salt until dough is smooth, scraping down side of bowl frequently with a rubber spatula.

2. Divide dough into 2 equal pieces. With palms of hands, roll each dough piece into a 10 × ¾-inch rope. Wrap and refrigerate for at least 3 hours or up to 3 days (or freeze for up to 6 months).

3. When ready to bake cookies, preheat oven to 350°F. Thinly slice dough crosswise to make ⅛-inch-thick rounds. Place cookies 1 inch apart on lightly greased cookie sheets. Bake 8 to 10 minutes, or until firm and very lightly browned on edges. Remove cookies to a rack and let cool completely. Store i ɔ a tightly covered container.

109 CHERRY SPIRALS

Prep: 20 minutes   Chill: 3 hours   Bake: 12 to 15 minutes
Makes: about 64

Dried sour cherries add an exciting tartness to these familiar cookies.
Look for the cherries in specialty food shops or see the mail-order source on
page 4.

½ cup dried sour cherries,
    finely chopped
½ cup walnuts, finely chopped
1 tablespoon granulated sugar
½ cup firmly packed brown
    sugar
1 stick (4 ounces) butter,
    softened

1 egg
1 teaspoon almond extract
1¾ cups flour
1 teaspoon baking powder
¼ teaspoon salt

1. In a small saucepan, combine dried cherries, walnuts, granulated sugar,
and ¼ cup water. Bring to a boil over high heat, stirring constantly to dissolve sugar. Reduce heat to medium and continue to boil, stirring, until mixture is thick, 3 to 5 minutes. Set filling aside.

2. In a large bowl, beat brown sugar and butter with an electric mixer on
medium speed until well blended. Beat in egg and almond extract until light
and fluffy. Beat in flour mixed with baking powder and salt until dough is
smooth, scraping down side of bowl frequently with a rubber spatula.

3. Between pieces of wax paper, roll dough out to make a 9 × 16-inch rectangle. Remove top piece of wax paper and spread dough with cherry-wal-
nut filling. Roll up dough jelly-roll fashion from a long side to make a
16-inch roll, removing bottom layer of wax paper as you roll. Cut roll in
half, wrap, and refrigerate at least 3 hours or up to 3 days (or freeze for up
to 6 months).

4. When ready to bake cookies, preheat oven to 350°F. Thinly slice dough
roll crosswise to make ¼-inch-thick cookies. Place cookies 2 inches apart on
lightly greased cookie sheets. Bake 12 to 15 minutes, or until firm and very
lightly browned on edges. Remove cookies to a rack and let cool completely.
Store in a tightly covered container.

110   BLACK WALNUT COOKIES

Prep: 10 minutes   Chill: 3 hours   Bake: 8 to 10 minutes
Makes: about 60

1 stick (4 ounces) butter,
   melted
½ cup granulated sugar
½ cup firmly packed brown
   sugar
1 egg

1 teaspoon vanilla extract
2¼ cups flour
½ teaspoon baking soda
¼ teaspoon salt
½ cup finely chopped black
   walnuts

1. In a large bowl, beat butter, granulated sugar, and brown sugar with an electric mixer on medium speed until well blended. Beat in egg and vanilla until light and fluffy.

2. Beat in flour mixed with baking soda and salt until dough is well blended, scraping down side of bowl frequently with a rubber spatula. Fold in black walnuts.

3. Divide dough into 2 pieces. With palms of hands, roll each dough piece to make a 2-inch-thick roll. Wrap and refrigerate at least 3 hours or up to 3 days (or freeze for up to 6 months).

4. When ready to bake cookies, preheat oven to 350°F. Thinly slice dough roll crosswise to make ⅛-inch-thick cookies. Place cookies 2 inches apart on lightly greased cookie sheets. Bake 8 to 10 minutes, or until firm and very lightly browned on edges. Remove cookies to a rack and let cool completely. Store in a tightly covered container.

111   CHOCOLATE COCONUT PINWHEELS

Prep: 20 minutes   Chill: 1½ hours   Bake: 8 to 10 minutes
Makes: about 48

1 stick (4 ounces) butter,
   softened
1 cup sugar
1 egg
1 teaspoon vanilla extract
2 cups cake flour

½ teaspoon baking soda
½ teaspoon salt
2 (1-ounce) squares
   unsweetened chocolate,
   melted
¾ cup flaked coconut

1. In a medium bowl, beat butter and sugar with an electric mixer on medium speed until light and fluffy. Beat in egg and vanilla.

2. Add cake flour mixed with baking soda and salt and beat until blended. Divide dough in half between 2 bowls. Blend melted chocolate into dough in one bowl; stir coconut into dough in other bowl. Cover each bowl with plastic wrap and refrigerate at least 1 hour, or until firm.

3. Gather chocolate dough into a ball; place between pieces of wax paper and roll out into an 8 × 12-inch rectangle. Repeat with coconut dough. Place one rectangle on top of the other and roll up from a long side into a 12-inch roll. Wrap in wax paper and refrigerate about 30 minutes, or until firm.

4. Preheat oven to 350°F. Using a sharp knife, cut dough into ¼-inch slices. Place about 3 inches apart on ungreased baking sheets. Bake 8 to 10 minutes, until lightly browned. Let cookies cool on sheets 2 minutes, then remove to a rack and let cool completely.

---

112 CHOCOLATE-WALNUT SLICES
Prep: 10 minutes   Chill: 3 hours   Bake: 10 to 12 minutes
Makes: about 66

Keep a roll of these in the freezer to bake in a hurry when unexpected guests arrive.

⅔ cup sugar
1 stick (4 ounces) butter, softened
1 egg
1 teaspoon vanilla extract
1⅓ cups flour

⅓ cup unsweetened cocoa powder
1 teaspoon baking powder
¼ teaspoon salt
½ cup finely chopped walnuts

1. In a large bowl, beat sugar and butter with an electric mixer on medium speed until well blended. Beat in egg and vanilla until light and fluffy.

2. Beat in flour mixed with cocoa, baking powder, and salt until dough is smooth, scraping down side of bowl frequently with a rubber spatula. Stir in nuts.

3. Divide dough into 2 equal pieces. With palms of hands, roll each dough piece into a 2-inch-thick roll. Wrap and refrigerate at least 3 hours or up to 3 days (or freeze for up to 6 months).

4. When ready to bake cookies, preheat oven to 350°F. Slice dough roll crosswise to make ⅛-inch-thick cookies. Place cookies 2 inches apart on lightly greased cookie sheets. Bake 10 to 12 minutes, or until firm. Remove cookies to a rack and let cool completely. Store in a tightly covered container.

113   CINNAMON 'N' SPICE SLICES
Prep: 10 minutes   Chill: 1 hour   Bake: 8 to 10 minutes
Makes: about 44

1 stick (4 ounces) butter, softened
½ cup firmly packed dark brown sugar
1 egg
1 teaspoon vanilla extract
1 cup flour
¼ cup finely ground almonds

¾ teaspoon cinnamon
½ teaspoon ground ginger
½ teaspoon ground allspice
½ teaspoon grated nutmeg
¼ teaspoon salt
⅓ cup powdered sugar
2 to 3 teaspoons orange juice

1. In a medium bowl, beat butter and brown sugar with an electric mixer on medium speed until light and fluffy. Beat in egg and vanilla until well blended.

2. Add flour mixed with almonds, cinnamon, ginger, allspice, nutmeg, and salt and beat until blended. Shape dough into 2 logs 8 inches long. Tightly wrap in wax paper and refrigerate at least 1 hour, until firm.

3. Preheat oven to 400°F. Cut logs into ⅜-inch-thick slices and place 2 inches apart on ungreased cookie sheets. Bake 8 to 10 minutes, or until bottoms begin to color. Let cookies cool on sheets 2 minutes, then remove to a rack and let cool completely.

4. In a small bowl, stir together powdered sugar and enough orange juice to make an icing of spreading consistency. Spread on completely cooled cookies.

114   CONNECTICUT YANKEE COOKIES
Prep: 10 minutes   Chill: 1 hour   Bake: 10 to 12 minutes
Makes: about 32

For a light, refreshing dessert, serve these nutmeg-flavored cookies with a bowl of sherbet.

1 stick (4 ounces) butter, softened
1½ ounces cream cheese, softened
½ cup firmly packed dark brown sugar

1 egg
½ teaspoon vanilla extract
1⅓ cups flour
¼ teaspoon salt
1 teaspoon grated nutmeg

1. In a medium bowl, beat butter, cream cheese, and brown sugar with an electric mixer on medium speed until light and fluffy. Beat in egg and vanilla until well blended.

2. Add flour mixed with salt and nutmeg and beat until well blended. Shape mixture into an 8-inch log. Wrap in wax paper and refrigerate 1 hour, until firm.

3. Preheat oven to 350°F. Using a sharp knife, cut dough into ¼-inch-thick slices. Place about 1 inch apart on ungreased baking sheets. Bake 10 to 12 minutes, until cookie edges begin to brown. Let cookies cool on sheets 2 minutes, then remove to a rack and let cool completely.

115 CORNMEAL ICEBOX COOKIES
Prep: 10 minutes   Chill: 3 hours   Bake: 10 to 12 minutes
Makes: about 60

You'll love the toasted cornmeal flavor of these delightful cookies.

1 cup sugar
1 stick (4 ounces) butter, softened
1 egg
1 teaspoon vanilla extract

1¼ cups flour
½ cup yellow cornmeal
1 teaspoon baking powder
¼ teaspoon salt

1. In a large bowl, beat sugar and butter with an electric mixer set on medium speed until well blended. Beat in egg and vanilla until light and fluffy.

2. Beat in flour mixed with cornmeal, baking powder, and salt until dough is smooth, scraping down side of bowl frequently with a rubber spatula.

3. Divide dough into 2 pieces. With palms of hands, roll each dough piece into a 2-inch-thick roll. Wrap and refrigerate for at least 3 hours or up to 3 days (or freeze for up to 6 months).

4. When ready to bake cookies, preheat oven to 350°F. Thinly slice dough roll crosswise to make ⅛-inch-thick cookies. Place cookies 2 inches apart on lightly greased cookie sheets.

5. Bake 10 to 12 minutes, or until firm and very lightly browned on edges. Remove cookies to a rack and let cool completely. Store in a tightly covered container.

116 GINGER SLICES
Prep: 10 minutes   Chill: 3 hours   Bake: 10 to 12 minutes
Makes: about 48

Crystallized ginger sets these easy-to-make cookies apart from the crowd.

1 cup sugar
1 stick (4 ounces) butter, softened
1 egg
1 teaspoon vanilla extract
1¾ cups flour

2 teaspoons ground ginger
1 teaspoon baking powder
¼ teaspoon salt
¼ cup finely chopped crystallized ginger

1. In a large bowl, beat sugar and butter with an electric mixer on medium speed until well blended. Beat in egg and vanilla until light and fluffy.

2. Beat in flour mixed with ground ginger, baking powder, and salt until dough is smooth, scraping down side of bowl frequently with a rubber spatula. Stir in crystallized ginger.

3. Divide dough into 2 pieces. With palms of hands, roll each dough piece to make a 2-inch-thick roll. Wrap and refrigerate for at least 3 hours or up to 3 days (or freeze for up to 6 months).

4. When ready to bake cookies, preheat oven to 350°F. Thinly slice dough roll crosswise to make ⅛-inch-thick cookies. Place cookies 2 inches apart on lightly greased cookie sheets. Bake 10 to 12 minutes, or until firm and very lightly browned on edges. Remove cookies to a rack and let cool completely. Store in a tightly covered container.

117 HAZELNUT BUTTER COOKIES
Prep: 15 minutes   Chill: 1 hour   Bake: 18 to 22 minutes
Makes: about 48

1 stick (4 ounces) plus 2 tablespoons butter, softened
1 cup powdered sugar
2 eggs
Pinch of salt

⅔ cup ground toasted hazelnuts
2 cups flour
2 tablespoons cornstarch
1 teaspoon vanilla extract
2 to 3 teaspoons fresh lemon juice

1. In a medium bowl, beat butter and ½ cup powdered sugar with an electric mixer on medium speed until light and fluffy. Beat in eggs, salt, and hazelnuts until well blended.

2. Add flour and cornstarch to sugar mixture and mix until blended. Divide dough in half. Roll each piece of dough into a 12-inch log. Tightly wrap in wax paper and refrigerate at least 1 hour, until firm.

3. Preheat oven to 350°F. Slice logs crosswise into ½-inch-thick cookies. Place 2 inches apart on greased cookie sheets. Bake 18 to 22 minutes, until bottoms begin to color. Let stand 2 minutes on cookie sheets, then remove to a wire rack and let cool completely.

4. In a small bowl, stir together remaining ½ cup powdered sugar, vanilla, and enough lemon juice to make an icing of spreading consistency. Spread icing over completely cooled cookies.

118 ICEBOX SAND TARTS

Prep: 10 minutes   Chill: 3 hours   Bake: 8 to 10 minutes
Makes: about 86

This sliced icebox version of these buttery cookies is much easier to make than the traditional paper-thin rolled version.

2 cups sugar	3 cups flour
2 eggs	1 teaspoon baking powder
2 sticks (8 ounces) butter, softened	1 teaspoon baking soda
1 teaspoon vanilla extract	¼ teaspoon salt
	½ teaspoon cinnamon

1. Set aside 2 tablespoons sugar. Separate 1 egg; cover and refrigerate yolk. In a large bowl, beat remaining sugar, egg white, remaining whole egg, butter, and vanilla with an electric mixer on medium speed until well blended.

2. Beat in flour mixed with baking powder, baking soda, and salt until dough is smooth, scraping down side of bowl frequently with a rubber spatula.

3. Divide dough into 2 pieces. With palms of hands, roll each dough piece into a log 2 inches thick. Wrap and refrigerate at least 3 hours, or overnight.

4. When ready to bake cookies, preheat oven to 350°F. Thinly slice dough roll crosswise to make paper-thin cookies. Place cookies 1 inch apart on lightly greased cookie sheets. Beat reserved yolk. With tip of a spoon, place a dot of egg yolk in center of each cookie. Combine reserved sugar and cinnamon; stir to mix well. Sprinkle a little cinnamon sugar onto each dab of egg yolk.

5. Bake 8 to 10 minutes, or until firm and very lightly browned around edges. Remove cookies to a rack and let cool completely. Store in a tightly covered container.

119   SPICY SHORTBREAD COOKIES

Prep: 5 minutes   Chill: 1 hour   Bake: 15 to 20 minutes
Makes: about 32

1 stick (4 ounces) butter, softened	1 teaspoon cinnamon
⅓ cup powdered sugar	½ teaspoon ground ginger
2 teaspoons grated lemon zest	¼ teaspoon ground allspice
1 cup flour	¼ teaspoon salt

1. In a medium bowl, beat butter and powdered sugar with an electric mixer on medium speed until light and fluffy. Beat in lemon zest. Add flour mixed with cinnamon, ginger, allspice, and salt and beat until blended.

2. Shape dough into an 8-inch log. Wrap tightly in wax paper and refrigerate at least 1 hour, until firm.

3. Preheat oven to 325°F. Using a sharp knife, cut dough into ¼-inch-thick slices. Place cookies about 1 inch apart on ungreased baking sheets. Bake 15 to 20 minutes, until pale golden, not brown. Let stand 2 minutes, then remove to a rack and let cool completely.

120   HAZELNUT SHORTBREAD COOKIES

Prep: 5 minutes   Chill: 1 hour   Bake: 15 to 20 minutes
Makes: about 32

¾ cup hazelnuts	2 teaspoons grated lemon zest
1 stick (4 ounces) butter, softened	1 cup flour
⅓ cup powdered sugar	¼ teaspoon cinnamon
	¼ teaspoon salt

1. Preheat oven to 350°F. Spread out nuts in a small baking dish and bake 5 to 7 minutes, or until dark outer skins are cracked and nuts are lightly browned. Finely chop hazelnuts.

2. In a medium bowl, beat butter and powdered sugar with an electric mixer on medium speed until light and fluffy. Beat in lemon zest. Add flour, ½ cup hazelnuts, cinnamon, and salt and beat until blended.

3. Shape dough into an 8-inch log. Roll log in remaining nuts. Tightly wrap in wax paper and refrigerate at least 1 hour, until firm.

4. Preheat oven to 325°F. Using a sharp knife, cut dough into ¼-inch-thick slices. Place about 1 inch apart on ungreased baking sheets. Bake 15 to 20 minutes, until pale golden, not brown. Let stand 2 minutes, then remove to a wire rack and let cool completely.

121 LEMON SLICES
Prep: 10 minutes   Chill: 1 hour   Bake: 10 to 12 minutes
Makes: about 64

2 sticks (8 ounces) butter, softened
1 (3-ounce) package cream cheese, softened
1 cup sugar
1 egg
½ teaspoon vanilla extract
½ teaspoon lemon extract
2½ cups flour
½ teaspoon salt
2 teaspoons grated lemon zest

1. In a medium bowl, beat butter, cream cheese, and sugar with an electric mixer on medium speed until light and fluffy. Beat in egg, vanilla, and lemon extract until blended.

2. Add flour, salt, and lemon zest and beat until well blended.

3. Divide dough in half. Shape each half into an 8-inch log. Wrap in floured wax paper and refrigerate 1 hour, or until firm.

4. Preheat oven to 350°F. Using a sharp knife, cut dough into ¼-inch-thick slices. Place about 1 inch apart on ungreased baking sheets. Bake 10 to 12 minutes, until cookie edges begin to brown. Let cookies cool on sheets 2 minutes, then remove to a rack and let cool completely.

122 LEMONY WONDERS
Prep: 10 minutes   Chill: 1 hour   Bake: 8 to 10 minutes
Makes: about 64

1½ sticks (6 ounces) butter, softened
⅔ cup powdered sugar
2 teaspoons lemon extract
2 teaspoons grated lemon zest
1¼ cups flour
½ cup cornstarch
2 to 3 teaspoons fresh lemon juice

1. In a medium bowl, beat butter and ⅓ cup powdered sugar with an electric mixer on medium speed until light and fluffy. Beat in lemon extract and 1 teaspoon lemon zest until well blended.

2. Beat flour and cornstarch into sugar mixture until blended. Shape dough into 2 logs 8 inches long. Tightly wrap in wax paper and refrigerate at least 1 hour, until firm.

3. Preheat oven to 350°F. Slice logs ¼ inch thick and place 2 inches apart on ungreased cookie sheets. Bake 8 to 10 minutes, until bottoms begin to color. Let stand 2 minutes on cookie sheets, then remove to a wire rack and let cool completely.

4. In a small bowl, stir remaining ⅓ cup powdered sugar with 1 teaspoon lemon zest and enough lemon juice to make an icing of spreading consistency. Spread icing over completely cooled cookies.

123 MINTY CHOCOLATE CRISPS
Prep: 10 minutes   Chill: 1 hour   Bake: 12 to 15 minutes
Makes: about 36

Chocolate mint lovers will find these wafers irresistible.

½ **cup solid vegetable shortening**	¾ **cup unsweetened cocoa powder**
1 **cup sugar**	½ **teaspoon baking soda**
1 **egg**	½ **teaspoon salt**
¼ **teaspoon peppermint extract**	⅓ **cup nonfat plain yogurt**
2 **cups flour**	

1. In a large bowl, beat shortening and sugar with an electric mixer on medium speed until light and fluffy. Beat in egg and peppermint extract until well blended.

2. Add flour mixed with cocoa, baking soda, and salt and beat until well blended. Stir in yogurt.

3. Shape mixture into an 8-inch log. Wrap in wax paper and refrigerate 1 hour, until firm.

4. Preheat oven to 350°F. Using a sharp knife, cut dough into ¼-inch-thick slices. Place about 1 inch apart on ungreased baking sheets. Bake 12 to 15 minutes, until cooked through. Let cookies cool on sheets 2 minutes, then remove to a rack and let cool completely.

124 NEAPOLITAN COOKIES
Prep: 15 minutes   Chill: 3 hours   Bake: 12 to 15 minutes
Makes: about 72

1 **cup sugar**	¼ **cup dried sour cherries, chopped**
1 **stick (4 ounces) butter, softened**	2 **to 3 drops of red food coloring (optional)**
2 **eggs**	1 **(1-ounce) square semisweet chocolate, melted**
1 **teaspoon vanilla extract**	2 **tablespoons semisweet mini chocolate chips**
2 **cups flour**	
1 **teaspoon baking powder**	
¼ **teaspoon salt**	
¼ **cup chopped blanched almonds**	

1. In a large bowl, beat sugar and butter with an electric mixer on medium speed until well blended. Beat in eggs and vanilla until light and fluffy.

2. Beat in flour mixed with baking powder and salt until dough is smooth, scraping down side of bowl frequently with a rubber spatula.

3. Divide dough into 3 pieces. Place one piece of dough in a small bowl; stir in almonds. Place a second piece of dough in another small bowl; stir in cherries and food coloring, if desired. Place the last piece of dough in a third small bowl; stir in melted chocolate and chocolate chips. Between pieces of wax paper, roll out each piece of dough to a 6-inch square. Wrap separately and refrigerate at least 3 hours or up to 3 days (or freeze for up to 6 months).

4. When ready to bake cookies, preheat oven to 350°F. Unwrap dough squares. Place squares one on top of another with chocolate in center. Slice dough crosswise to make three 2-inch-wide stacks of dough. Cut each stack crosswise to make ¼-inch-thick cookies.

5. Place cookies 2 inches apart on lightly greased cookie sheets. Bake 12 to 15 minutes, or until firm and very lightly browned on edges. Remove cookies to a rack and let cool completely. Store in a tightly covered container.

---

125 OATMEAL ICEBOX COOKIES
Prep: 10 minutes   Chill: 3 hours   Bake: 12 to 15 minutes
Makes: about 60

We like to use old-fashioned rolled oats for these because they make crunchier cookies.

¾ cup firmly packed brown sugar	1 cup flour
1 stick (4 ounces) butter, softened	1½ cups rolled oats
	1 teaspoon baking powder
1 egg	¼ teaspoon salt
1 teaspoon vanilla extract	½ cup chopped walnuts
	Cinnamon

1. In a large bowl, beat brown sugar and butter with an electric mixer on medium speed until well blended. Beat in egg and vanilla until light and fluffy.

2. Beat in flour mixed with oatmeal, baking powder, and salt until dough is smooth, scraping down side of bowl frequently with a rubber spatula. Fold in walnuts.

3. Divide dough into 2 pieces. With palms of hands, roll each dough piece to make a 2-inch-thick roll. Wrap and refrigerate at least 3 hours or up to 3 days (or freeze for up to 6 months).

4. When ready to bake cookies, preheat oven to 350°F. Slice dough roll crosswise to make ¼-inch-thick cookies. Place cookies 2 inches apart on lightly greased cookie sheets. Sprinkle tops lightly with cinnamon. Bake 12 to 15 minutes, or until firm and very lightly browned on edges. Remove cookies to a rack and let cool completely. Store in a tightly covered container.

126   ZEBRA COOKIES
Prep: 15 minutes   Chill: 3 hours   Bake: 12 to 15 minutes
Makes: about 48

Crisp and buttery, these cookies are worth their stripes.

⅔ cup sugar
1 stick (4 ounces) butter,
   softened
1 egg
2 teaspoons vanilla extract
1¾ cups flour

½ teaspoon baking powder
¼ teaspoon salt
2 (1-ounce) squares
   unsweetened chocolate,
   melted

1. In a large bowl, beat sugar and butter with an electric mixer on medium speed until well blended. Beat in egg and vanilla until light and fluffy.

2. Beat in flour mixed with baking powder and salt until dough is smooth, scraping down side of bowl frequently with a rubber spatula.

3. Divide dough in half. Remove one half of dough and shape into a *square* roll 2 inches to a side; be sure to make sides flat. Place remaining dough in a small bowl. With a fork, stir in chocolate until well blended. Shape chocolate dough into a square roll, 2 inches to a side. Wrap and refrigerate at least 3 hours or up to 3 days (or freeze for up to 6 months).

4. When ready to bake cookies, preheat oven to 350°F. Slice both pieces of dough lengthwise to make 4 long slices. Reassemble rolls alternating chocolate and light doughs. Slice rolls crosswise to make ¼-inch-thick cookies. Place cookies 2 inches apart on lightly greased cookie sheets. Bake 12 to 15 minutes, or until firm and very lightly browned on edges. Remove cookies to a rack and let cool completely. Store in a tightly covered container.

127   SUNFLOWER SLICES
Prep: 10 minutes   Chill: 2 hours   Bake: 10 to 12 minutes
Makes: about 36

The crunch of sunflower kernels adds interest to these buttery icebox cookies.

1 stick (4 ounces) butter,
   softened
⅓ cup sugar
1 egg

1 teaspoon vanilla extract
1¼ cups flour
⅓ cup shelled sunflower seeds
   (kernels)

1. In a large bowl, beat butter and sugar with an electric mixer on medium speed until well blended. Beat in egg and vanilla until light and fluffy.

2. Add flour and beat until dough is smooth, scraping down side of bowl frequently with a rubber spatula. Stir in sunflower kernels.

3. Divide dough in half. With palms of hands, roll each dough piece into a 2-inch-thick roll. Wrap and refrigerate 2 to 3 hours, until firm, or up to 3 days (or freeze for up to 6 months).

4. When ready to bake cookies, preheat oven to 350°F. Slice dough roll crosswise to make ¼-inch-thick cookies. Place cookies 2 inches apart on lightly greased cookie sheets. Bake 10 to 12 minutes, or until firm. Remove cookies to a rack and let cool completely. Store in a tightly covered container.

128 PEACH BLOSSOMS
Prep: 15 minutes   Chill: 3 hours   Bake: 12 to 15 minutes
Makes: about 32

Designed to resemble the peach-colored peanut butter candies we find in stores around the holidays, these cookies really have peaches in them.

½ cup sugar	1 teaspoon baking powder
1 stick (4 ounces) butter, softened	¼ teaspoon salt
1 egg	¼ cup finely chopped dried peaches
1 teaspoon vanilla extract	¼ cup chunky peanut butter
1¾ cups flour	

1. In a large bowl, beat sugar and butter with an electric mixer on medium speed until well blended. Beat in egg and vanilla until light and fluffy.

2. Beat in flour mixed with baking powder and salt until dough is smooth, scraping down sides of bowl frequently with a rubber scraper.

3. Divide dough into 2 pieces. Place one piece of dough in a small bowl; stir in peaches. Set aside. Place second piece of dough in another small bowl; stir in peanut butter. Between pieces of wax paper, roll out peach dough to a 7 × 8-inch rectangle. With palms of hands, roll peanut butter dough to make an 8-inch roll. Remove top piece of wax paper from peach dough. Place peanut butter dough roll on top of peach dough rectangle and roll up peach dough around it to make an 8-inch-long roll. Wrap and refrigerate at least 3 hours or up to 3 days (or freeze for up to 6 months).

4. When ready to bake cookies, preheat oven to 350°F. Slice dough roll crosswise to make ¼-inch-thick cookies. Place cookies 2 inches apart on lightly greased cookie sheets. Bake 12 to 15 minutes, or until firm and very lightly browned on edges. Remove cookies to a rack and let cool completely. Store in a tightly covered container.

129   WALNUT WAFERS
Prep: 10 minutes   Chill: 1 hour   Bake: 10 to 12 minutes
Makes: about 32

1 stick (4 ounces) butter,
   softened
⅓ cup firmly packed dark
   brown sugar
1 teaspoon vanilla extract

1 cup flour
½ teaspoon baking powder
¾ cup toasted walnuts, finely
   chopped

1. In a large bowl, beat butter with an electric mixer on medium speed until creamy. Add brown sugar and vanilla. Continue to beat until light and fluffy. In a small bowl, stir together flour and baking powder. Gradually blend into butter-sugar mixture. Stir in ½ cup walnuts. Shape mixture into an 8-inch log. Roll log in remaining walnuts to coat. Wrap in wax paper and refrigerate 1 hour or freeze until firm.

2. Preheat oven to 350°F. Using a sharp knife, cut dough into ¼-inch-thick slices. Place about 1 inch apart on ungreased baking sheets. Bake 10 to 12 minutes, until lightly browned. Using a wide spatula, remove to a rack to cool.

Chapter 5

In the Chips

Ask almost anyone what their favorite cookie is, and they will say, "chocolate chip." Chocolate chip cookies are so popular that all across America there are whole stores devoted to producing them. Chances are the first cookie recipe you ever made had chocolate chips in it, and the recipe you make most frequently has chocolate chips in it. For this reason —and also by request from our children—we decided to devote a whole chapter to chocolate chip cookies.

Whether you drop them, roll them, shape them, or bake them into bars, chocolate chip cookies offer something extra to cookie munchers. That aromatic, silky smooth, not-too-sweet, perky little nugget of melt-in-your-mouth goodness makes any cookie it snuggles into the first to disappear from the cookie platter. What a wonder, then, that someone didn't think of making them until the 1930s.

Chocolate chips first appeared on the market in 1939, just in time to lift the nation's spirits from depression. After several years of printing Mrs. Ruth Wakefield's recipe for Toll House Cookies on the wrapper of their semisweet chocolate bars, the Nestlé Company began producing uniformly shaped little drops of chocolate especially formulated to keep their shape during baking yet remain smooth textured for perfect eating. The rest is history, and today the original chips have been joined by miniature chips, butterscotch chips, peanut butter chips, mint chocolate chips, and white baking chips. (By the way, you'll find the original Toll House Cookie in "American Classics" on page 159.)

The possibilities for using chips in cookie recipes are endless. Once you have explored our collection of chip-full recipes, you might want to add some chips to recipes in other chapters. Our only discovery in testing this chapter was that no matter how good we thought a chopped candy bar would be in a recipe, the specially formulated chips were usually better. Chocolate bars were created to be enjoyed cool and right from the wrapper; the baking performance of different brands of eating chocolate varies greatly, and sometimes the smooth creamy chocolate that went into the oven comes out crisp and crunchy after baking.

We hope you will have as much fun tasting this chapter as we had testing it. We enjoyed every last chip of it!

130   BRICKLE CHOCOLATE CHIP BARS
Prep: 10 minutes   Bake: 15 to 20 minutes   Makes: 24

2 sticks (8 ounces) butter,
    softened
1 cup firmly packed dark
    brown sugar
1 egg
1 teaspoon vanilla extract

2 cups flour
  Pinch of salt
1 (6-ounce) package Bits
    'O Brickle
½ cup semisweet chocolate
    chips

1. Preheat oven to 350°F. In a medium bowl, beat butter and brown sugar with an electric mixer on medium speed until light and fluffy. Beat in egg and vanilla.

2. Add flour and salt and beat until blended. Stir in brickle and chocolate chips. Press into an ungreased 9 × 13-inch pan.

3. Bake 15 to 20 minutes, until edges brown. Remove pan to a rack and let cool 5 minutes before cutting into 24 bars.

---

131   CHOCOLATE CHIP DREAMS
Prep: 20 minutes   Bake: 11 to 13 minutes   Makes: about 36

These are not mere chocolate chip cookies, but cookies with grated chocolate in the batter. They're irresistible—especially while still warm.

2 cups all-purpose flour
½ cup oat flour (see Note)
1 teaspoon baking powder
1 teaspoon baking soda
½ teaspoon salt
1 stick (4 ounces) butter,
    softened
½ cup shortening
1 cup granulated sugar

1 cup firmly packed dark
    brown sugar
2 eggs
1 teaspoon vanilla extract
12 ounces semisweet chocolate
    chips (2 cups)
4 (1-ounce) squares semisweet
    chocolate, grated

1. Preheat oven to 350°F. In a small bowl, stir together flour, oat flour, baking powder, baking soda, and salt.

2. In a large bowl, beat butter, shortening, granulated sugar, and dark brown sugar with an electric mixer on medium speed until creamy. Beat in eggs and vanilla until well blended.

3. Add flour mixture and beat until well blended. Mix in chocolate chips and grated chocolate.

4. Place golf ball–sized balls 2½ inches apart on ungreased cookie sheets. Bake 11 to 13 minutes, or until lightly browned. Let stand 2 minutes on cookie sheets, then remove to a rack and let cool completely.

NOTE: *To make ½ cup oat flour, finely grind 1 cup oatmeal in a food processor or blender.*

132 BANANA CHOCOLATE CHIP COOKIES
Prep: 10 minutes   Bake: 8 to 10 minutes   Makes: about 32

2 sticks (8 ounces) unsalted butter, softened	2 cups flour
1½ cups powdered sugar	1 teaspoon baking powder
½ teaspoon lemon extract	½ teaspoon salt
½ cup mashed banana (about 1 medium)	6 ounces semisweet mini chocolate chips (1 cup)

1. Preheat oven to 400°F. In a medium bowl, beat butter and powdered sugar with an electric mixer on medium speed until creamy. Beat in lemon extract and mashed banana until well blended.

2. Add flour mixed with baking powder and salt and beat until blended. Stir in the chocolate chips.

3. Drop heaping teaspoonfuls of dough 2 inches apart on greased cookie sheets. Bake 8 to 10 minutes, just until edges start to brown. Let stand 2 minutes on cookie sheets, then remove to a rack and let cool completely.

---

133 GIANT DOUBLE CHOCOLATE CHIP COOKIES
Prep: 15 minutes   Bake: 15 to 18 minutes   Makes: 15

1 stick (4 ounces) butter, softened	1½ teaspoons vanilla extract
1 cup firmly packed dark brown sugar	1½ cups flour
2 (1-ounce) squares unsweetened chocolate, melted	½ teaspoon baking powder
	½ teaspoon baking soda
	¼ teaspoon salt
2 eggs	12 ounces semisweet chocolate chips (2 cups)
	½ cup chopped walnuts

1. Preheat oven to 350°F. In a medium bowl, beat butter and brown sugar with an electric mixer on medium speed until creamy. Beat in melted chocolate, eggs, and vanilla.

2. Mix together flour, baking powder, baking soda, and salt. Beat into chocolate mixture until well blended. Stir in chocolate chips and walnuts.

3. Drop by ¼-cupfuls 3 inches apart onto greased cookie sheets; flatten gently. Bake 15 to 18 minutes, until lightly browned around edges. Let cookies cool on sheets 3 minutes, then remove to a rack and let cool completely.

134   BANANA CHOCONUT COOKIES
Prep: 10 minutes   Bake: 12 to 15 minutes   Makes: about 48

2 sticks (8 ounces) unsalted butter, softened
1½ cups firmly packed dark brown sugar
1 egg
2 teaspoons banana extract or 1 tablespoon banana liqueur
¾ cup mashed banana (about 1 large)
2½ cups flour
1 teaspoon baking powder
½ teaspoon salt
12 ounces semisweet mini chocolate chips (2 cups)
½ cup chopped pecans

1. Preheat oven to 325°F. In a medium bowl, beat butter and brown sugar with an electric mixer on medium speed until creamy. Beat in egg, banana extract, and banana until well blended.

2. Add flour mixed with baking powder and salt to sugar mixture and beat until blended. Stir in the chocolate chips and nuts.

3. Place teaspoonfuls of dough 2 inches apart on ungreased cookie sheets. Bake 12 to 15 minutes, just until edges start to brown. Remove to a rack and let cool completely.

135   CHOCOLATE CHOCOLATE CHIP CRACKLES
Prep: 10 minutes   Chill: 1 hour   Bake: 10 to 12 minutes   Makes: about 36

2 cups flour
⅔ cup unsweetened cocoa powder
2 teaspoons baking powder
½ teaspoon salt
1½ sticks (6 ounces) butter, softened
2 cups sugar
4 eggs
2 teaspoons vanilla extract
12 ounces semisweet chocolate chips (2 cups)

1. In a small bowl, stir together flour, cocoa, baking powder, and salt.

2. In a large bowl, beat butter and sugar with an electric mixer on medium speed until creamy. Beat in eggs, one at a time, and vanilla. Add flour mixture and beat until well blended. Stir in the chocolate chips. Cover and refrigerate until well chilled, at least 1 hour, or overnight.

3. Preheat oven to 350°F. Drop dough by heaping teaspoonfuls 2 inches apart onto greased cookie sheets. Bake 10 to 12 minutes, or until dry and set. Let stand 2 minutes, then remove to a rack and let cool completely.

136   CRANBERRY CHOCOLATE CHIP COOKIES
Prep: 10 minutes   Bake: 12 to 15 minutes   Makes: about 30

1 stick (4 ounces) butter,
   softened
¾ cup firmly packed dark
   brown sugar
1 egg
½ teaspoon vanilla extract
1 cup flour
½ teaspoon baking powder

¼ teaspoon salt
½ cup dried cranberries (about
   2 ounces), chopped
½ cup semisweet chocolate
   chips
½ cup chopped walnuts

1. Preheat oven to 350°F. In a medium bowl, beat butter and brown sugar with an electric mixer on medium speed until creamy. Beat in egg and vanilla until well blended.

2. Add flour mixed with baking powder and salt and beat until blended. Stir in dried cranberries, chocolate chips, and walnuts.

3. Drop by teaspoonfuls 2 inches apart onto greased cookie sheets. Bake 12 to 15 minutes. Let cookies cool on sheets 2 minutes, then remove to a rack and let cool completely.

137   CREAMY CHOCOLATE CHIP DROPS
Prep: 10 minutes   Bake: 20 to 25 minutes   Makes: about 48

1½ sticks (6 ounces) butter,
   softened
1 (3-ounce) package cream
   cheese, softened
¾ cup granulated sugar
1 teaspoon vanilla extract

2 cups cake flour
¼ teaspoon salt
¾ cup finely chopped
   semisweet chocolate
   chips
½ cup powdered sugar

1. Preheat oven to 300°F. In a medium bowl, beat butter, cream cheese, and granulated sugar with an electric mixer on medium speed until light and fluffy. Beat in vanilla.

2. Add cake flour and salt and beat until blended. Stir in chocolate chips.

3. Drop by teaspoonfuls 2 inches apart onto ungreased cookie sheets. Bake 20 to 25 minutes, until set but not browned. Let cookies cool on sheets 2 minutes. Roll in powdered sugar, transfer to a rack, and let cool completely.

138   CHOCOLATE CHUNK BUTTERSCOTCH COOKIES

Prep: 10 minutes   Bake: 7 to 9 minutes   Makes: 24

2 sticks (8 ounces) unsalted
   butter, softened
1 cup firmly packed dark
   brown sugar
1 egg
1 teaspoon vanilla extract

½ teaspoon salt
1¾ cups flour
1½ cups semisweet chocolate
   chunks (9 ounces), very
   coarsely chopped

1. Preheat oven to 400°F. In a medium bowl, beat butter and brown sugar with an electric mixer on medium speed until creamy. Beat in egg, vanilla, and salt until well blended.

2. Add flour and beat until blended. Stir in chopped chocolate. Drop heaping teaspoons of dough 2 inches apart onto greased cookie sheets.

3. Bake 7 to 9 minutes, just until edges start to brown. Let stand 2 minutes on cookie sheets, then remove to a rack and let cool completely.

139   CHOCOLATE CHIP GRANOLA BARS

Prep: 8 minutes   Bake: 20 to 25 minutes   Makes: 24

Our family and friends have nicknamed these "Ooey-Gooey Bars."

1 stick (4 ounces) butter,
   softened
¼ cup firmly packed dark
   brown sugar
¼ cup honey
1 teaspoon vanilla extract

2 cups flour
1 teaspoon baking soda
   Pinch of salt
2 cups granola
6 ounces semisweet chocolate
   chips (1 cup)

1. Preheat oven to 350°F. Grease a 9-inch square pan. In a medium bowl, beat butter, brown sugar, and honey with an electric mixer on medium speed until light and fluffy. Beat in vanilla.

2. Add flour mixed with baking soda and salt and beat until blended. Stir in granola and chocolate chips. Press into prepared pan.

3. Bake 20 to 25 minutes, or until edges brown. Remove pan to a rack and let cool completely before cutting into 24 bars.

140 CHOCOLATE CHUNK LEMON DREAMS
Prep: 10 minutes   Bake: 7 to 9 minutes   Makes: 24

2 sticks (8 ounces) unsalted
  butter, softened
½ cup firmly packed dark
  brown sugar
¼ cup plus 2 tablespoons
  granulated sugar
1 egg
1 tablespoon grated lemon
  zest

1 teaspoon vanilla extract
½ teaspoon lemon extract
½ teaspoon salt
1¾ cups flour
1½ cups semisweet chocolate
  chunks (9 ounces),
  roughly chopped

1. Preheat oven to 400°F. In a medium bowl, beat butter, brown sugar, and granulated sugar with an electric mixer on medium speed until creamy. Beat in egg, lemon zest, vanilla, lemon extract, and salt until well blended.

2. Add flour and beat until blended. Stir in chopped chocolate. Drop dough by heaping teaspoons 2 inches apart on greased cookie sheets.

3. Bake 7 to 9 minutes, just until edges start to brown. Let stand 2 minutes on cookie sheets, then remove to a rack and let cool completely.

---

141 MACADAMIA-CHIP COOKIES
Prep: 10 minutes   Bake: 12 to 15 minutes   Makes: about 34

Because it is difficult to find unsalted macadamia nuts in many parts of the country, we did not include salt in this dough. The salt remaining on the nuts is just enough to balance the dough's sweetness.

1 stick (4 ounces) butter,
  softened
⅓ cup powdered sugar
⅓ cup firmly packed brown
  sugar
1 egg
1 teaspoon vanilla extract

1½ cups flour
2 teaspoons baking powder
½ cup salted macadamia nuts
½ cup white baking chips
½ cup semisweet chocolate
  chips

1. Preheat oven to 350°F. In a large bowl, beat butter, powdered sugar, and brown sugar with an electric mixer on medium speed until well blended. Beat in egg and vanilla until light and fluffy.

2. Beat in flour mixed with baking powder until dough is smooth, scraping down side of bowl frequently with a rubber spatula. Place macadamia nuts in a strainer and shake to remove excess salt. Fold macadamia nuts, white chocolate chips, and semisweet chocolate chips into dough.

3. Drop by heaping teaspoonfuls 2 inches apart onto lightly greased cookie sheets. Bake 12 to 15 minutes, or until golden brown. Let cookies cool 2 minutes on sheets, then remove to racks and let cool completely. Store in a tightly covered container.

142   CHOCOLATE MARSHMALLOW BOMBS
Prep: 10 minutes   Bake: 12 to 15 minutes   Makes: about 30

1 stick (4 ounces) butter, softened
1 cup sugar
1 egg
1 teaspoon vanilla extract
1½ cups flour
⅓ cup unsweetened cocoa powder

½ teaspoon baking soda
½ teaspoon salt
6 ounces semisweet mini chocolate chips (1 cup)
½ cup mini marshmallows, frozen

1. Preheat oven to 375°F. In a large bowl, beat butter and sugar with an electric mixer on medium speed until creamy. Beat in egg and vanilla.

2. Add flour mixed with cocoa powder, baking soda, and salt and beat until blended. Stir in chocolate chips.

3. Shape dough into 1-inch balls around a few marshmallows, pinching ends of dough to enclose marshmallows completely. Place 1 inch apart on ungreased cookie sheets. Bake 12 to 15 minutes, until set. Let stand 2 minutes, then remove to a rack and let cool completely.

143   MINT CHOCOLATE CHIP COOKIES
Prep: 10 minutes   Bake: 8 to 10 minutes   Makes: about 36

These cookies are designed for the ardent chocolate-mint lovers.

1 stick (4 ounces) plus 2 tablespoons butter, softened
1 cup firmly packed dark brown sugar
1 egg
¼ cup plain nonfat yogurt
½ teaspoon vanilla extract

½ teaspoon mint extract
1¾ cups flour
½ cup unsweetened cocoa powder
½ teaspoon baking soda
½ teaspoon salt
6 ounces semisweet mini chocolate chips (1 cup)

1. Preheat oven to 400°F. In a large bowl, beat butter and brown sugar with an electric mixer on medium speed until creamy. Beat in egg, yogurt, vanilla, and mint extract until well blended.

2. Add flour mixed with cocoa powder, baking soda, and salt and beat until well blended. Stir in chocolate chips.

3. Drop by teaspoonfuls onto greased cookie sheets. Bake 8 to 10 minutes. Let cookies cool on sheets 2 minutes, then remove to a rack and let cool completely.

144 NUTTY CHOCONUT BARS
Prep: 10 minutes   Bake: 20 to 25 minutes   Makes: 20

¾ cup firmly packed dark
   brown sugar
2 eggs
1 teaspoon vanilla extract
½ cup whole wheat flour
¼ teaspoon baking soda

¼ teaspoon salt
⅔ cup semisweet chocolate
   chips
⅔ cup flaked coconut
⅔ cup chopped walnuts

1. Preheat oven to 350°F. Grease an 8-inch square pan. In a large bowl, beat brown sugar, eggs, and vanilla with an electric mixer on medium speed until well blended.

2. Add whole wheat flour mixed with baking soda and salt and beat until blended. Stir in chocolate chips, coconut, and walnuts. Turn batter into prepared pan, leveling surface.

3. Bake 20 to 25 minutes, until a toothpick inserted in center comes out clean. Remove to a rack. Let cool completely in pan before cutting into 20 bars.

145 CHOCOLATE CHIP NUTTY OATDROPS
Prep: 10 minutes   Bake: 8 to 10 minutes   Makes: about 36

1½ sticks (6 ounces) butter,
   softened
½ cup firmly packed dark
   brown sugar
¼ cup granulated sugar
1½ cups rolled oats

¾ cup flour
1 teaspoon baking powder
½ teaspoon salt
6 ounces semisweet chocolate
   chips (1 cup)
¾ cup flaked coconut, toasted

1. Preheat oven to 350°F. In a large bowl, beat butter, brown sugar, and granulated sugar with an electric mixer on medium speed until creamy. Add oatmeal mixed into flour, baking powder, and salt and stir until well blended. Mix in chocolate chips and coconut.

2. Place golf ball–sized rounds 2½ inches apart on ungreased cookie sheets. Bake 8 to 10 minutes, until browned around edges. Let stand 2 minutes on cookie sheets, then remove to a rack and let cool completely.

146   CHOCOLATE CHIP OATMEAL COOKIES
Prep: 10 minutes   Bake: 10 to 12 minutes   Makes: about 36

¾ cup flour
1½ cups rolled oats
½ teaspoon baking soda
½ teaspoon salt
1 stick (4 ounces) butter,
  softened
½ cup granulated sugar
½ cup firmly packed dark
  brown sugar

1 egg
½ teaspoon vanilla extract
1 tablespoon Kahlúa or other
  coffee-flavored liqueur
6 ounces semisweet chocolate
  chips (1 cup)

1. Preheat oven to 350°F. In a small bowl, stir together flour, oatmeal, baking soda, and salt.

2. In a large bowl, beat butter, granulated sugar, and brown sugar with an electric mixer on medium speed until creamy. Beat in egg, vanilla, and Kahlúa until well blended. Add flour mixture and beat until well blended. Stir in chocolate chips.

3. Drop dough by teaspoonfuls 2 inches apart onto greased cookie sheets. Bake 10 to 12 minutes. Let stand 2 minutes, then remove to a rack and let cool completely.

147   ORANGE CHOCOLATE CHIP SHORTBREAD SQUARES
Prep: 7 minutes   Bake: 25 to 30 minutes   Makes: 25

The combination of chocolate and orange makes these quick-to-create bars irresistible.

1 stick (4 ounces) butter,
  softened
⅓ cup plus 2 teaspoons sugar
2 teaspoons orange-flavored
  liqueur

1 cup flour
¼ teaspoon salt
2 teaspoons grated orange zest
½ cup semisweet mini
  chocolate chips

1. Preheat oven to 325°F. In a medium bowl, beat butter and ⅓ cup sugar with an electric mixer on medium speed until light and fluffy. Beat in orange liqueur.

2. Add flour, salt, and orange zest and beat until blended. Stir in chocolate chips.

3. Press dough evenly over bottom of an ungreased 9-inch square pan. Bake 25 to 30 minutes, until golden. Remove from oven and sprinkle 2 teaspoons sugar over top. Remove pan to a rack, cut into 25 squares while hot, and let cool completely.

148 PEANUT BUTTER CHOCOLATE CHIP COOKIES

Prep: 15 minutes   Chill: 2 hours   Bake: 8 to 10 minutes
Makes: about 36

1 cup firmly packed light brown sugar
1 stick (4 ounces) butter, softened
½ cup chunky peanut butter
1 egg

1½ cups flour
1 teaspoon baking soda
½ teaspoon baking powder
½ teaspoon salt
1½ cups semisweet chocolate chips (9 ounces)

1. In a large bowl, beat brown sugar, butter, peanut butter, and egg with an electric mixer on medium speed until well blended.

2. In a small bowl, stir together flour, baking soda, baking powder, and salt. Add to butter-sugar mixture and beat until blended. Stir in chocolate chips. Cover and refrigerate until well chilled, about 2 hours or overnight.

3. Preheat oven to 375°F. Shape chilled dough into 1¼-inch balls and place 3 inches apart on ungreased cookie sheets. Flatten in crisscross pattern with tines of a fork. Bake 8 to 10 minutes. Let stand 2 minutes, then remove to a rack and let cool completely.

149 CHOCOLATE PECAN BARS

Prep: 10 minutes   Bake: 25 to 30 minutes   Makes: 25

1 stick (4 ounces) butter, softened
¼ cup plus 2 tablespoons firmly packed dark brown sugar
1 egg
1 teaspoon vanilla extract

2 teaspoons grated lemon zest
¾ cup finely chopped pecans
1 cup plus 1 tablespoon flour
¼ teaspoon salt
¾ cup semisweet chocolate chips

1. Preheat oven to 350°F. In a medium bowl, beat butter and ¼ cup brown sugar with an electric mixer on medium speed until creamy. Beat in egg, vanilla, and lemon zest until blended.

2. Add ½ cup pecans, ¾ cup plus 2 tablespoons flour, and salt and beat until dough forms. Using a spoon because dough will be sticky, press two thirds into bottom of an 8-inch square pan. Sprinkle chocolate chips evenly over dough.

3. To dough remaining in bowl, add 2 tablespoons brown sugar and remaining 3 tablespoons flour. Crumble brown sugar mixture over chocolate chips, then sprinkle with remaining ¼ cup chopped pecans. Press brown sugar mixture and nuts gently into dough.

4. Bake 25 to 30 minutes, until light brown and set. Remove to a rack and let cool thoroughly before cutting into 25 bars.

150 CHOCOLATE CHIP PALMIERS

Prep: 10 minutes   Chill: 15 minutes   Bake: 20 minutes
Makes: about 40

These quick-to-make pastries look store-bought and taste even better.

½ (17¼-ounce) package frozen
  puff pastry sheets
¾ cup sugar

4 tablespoons butter, softened
¾ cup semisweet mini
  chocolate chips

1. Thaw puff pastry according to package directions.

2. Sprinkle ½ cup sugar over work surface. Place 1 sheet of puff pastry over sugar and sprinkle remaining ¼ cup sugar on top. With a rolling pin, roll dough into an 11 × 14-inch rectangle. Spread softened butter over dough and sprinkle chocolate chips on top. With heel of hand, gently press chips into surface of dough.

3. Fold each long side of dough into center, so sides almost meet. Fold again, to bring folded edges together. Pastry should be 4 layers thick. Cover with plastic wrap and refrigerate 15 minutes.

4. Preheat oven to 400°F. Place one ungreased cookie sheet on top of another to create a double-insulated pan. Line top cookie sheet with parchment paper or foil.

5. Using a very sharp knife, cut pastry ¼ inch thick and place slices 1 inch apart on prepared cookie sheet. Bake 15 minutes. Turn over each palmier and bake 5 minutes longer, or until golden brown. Remove to a wire rack and let cool completely before serving.

151 PUFFED WHEAT CHIPPIES

Prep: 10 minutes   Bake: 10 to 12 minutes   Makes: about 54

⅔ cup solid vegetable
  shortening
½ cup sugar
1 egg
2 teaspoons vanilla extract
1 cup flour

½ teaspoon baking powder
¼ teaspoon salt
2 cups puffed wheat cereal
½ cup semisweet chocolate
  chips
½ cup milk chocolate chips

1. Preheat oven to 350°F. In a large bowl, beat shortening and sugar with an electric mixer on medium speed until well blended. Beat in egg and vanilla until light and fluffy.

2. Add flour mixed with baking powder and salt and beat until dough is smooth, scraping down sides of bowl frequently with a rubber scraper. Fold in cereal, semisweet chocolate chips, and milk chocolate chips.

3. Drop by heaping teaspoonfuls 2 inches apart onto lightly greased cookie sheets. Bake 10 to 12 minutes, or until edges are golden brown. Let cookies cool 2 minutes on sheets, then remove to racks and let cool completely. Store in a tightly covered container.

152 CHOCOLATE CHIP PUMPKIN DROPS

Prep: 15 minutes   Bake: 8 to 10 minutes   Makes: about 60

1 stick (4 ounces) butter, softened
1½ cups firmly packed dark brown sugar
1 cup canned pumpkin puree
1 egg
2 teaspoons grated orange zest
½ teaspoon orange extract
2¾ cups flour
2 teaspoons baking powder
1 teaspoon baking soda
1 teaspoon cinnamon
½ teaspoon grated nutmeg
½ teaspoon ground ginger
½ teaspoon salt
¾ cup semisweet chocolate chips
¾ cup chopped walnuts

1. Preheat oven to 400°F. In a medium bowl, beat butter and brown sugar with an electric mixer on medium speed until creamy. Beat in pumpkin, egg, orange zest, and orange extract.

2. Mix together flour, baking powder, baking soda, cinnamon, nutmeg, ginger, and salt. Add to pumpkin mixture and beat until well blended. Stir in chocolate chips and walnuts.

3. Drop by heaping teaspoonfuls 2 inches apart onto ungreased cookie sheets. Bake 8 to 10 minutes, or until lightly browned around edges. Let cookies cool on sheets 2 minutes, then remove to a rack and let cool completely.

153 CHOCOLATE CHIP SHORTBREAD

Prep: 5 minutes   Bake: 20 to 25 minutes   Makes: 12

1 stick (4 ounces) butter, softened
¼ cup powdered sugar
1 teaspoon grated orange zest
½ teaspoon vanilla extract
2 cups flour
¼ teaspoon salt
½ cup semisweet mini chocolate chips
2 tablespoons granulated sugar

1. Preheat oven to 325°F. In a medium bowl, beat butter and powdered sugar with an electric mixer on medium speed until light and fluffy. Add orange zest and vanilla. Stir in flour and salt until blended. Stir in chocolate chips.

2. Squeeze dough into a ball. On an ungreased cookie sheet press ball into an 8-inch disk about ½ inch thick. Crimp edges and prick all over with fork. Using a knife, score into 12 wedges.

3. Bake 20 to 25 minutes, or until golden but not brown. Sprinkle granulated sugar over top. Let cool in pan on a wire rack 5 minutes. Then cut into wedges and let cookies cool completely on rack.

154 CRUNCHY CHOCOLATE CHIP SHORTBREAD DROPS

Prep: 10 minutes   Bake: 35 to 40 minutes   Makes: about 36

The long slow baking makes these chocolatey cookies crunchy and irresistible.

2 sticks (8 ounces) butter, softened	½ teaspoon baking powder
¾ cup powdered sugar	¼ teaspoon salt
1 teaspoon vanilla extract	6 ounces semisweet chocolate
2 cups cake flour	chips (1 cup)
	½ cup chopped walnuts

1. Preheat oven to 300°F. In a medium bowl, beat butter and powdered sugar with an electric mixer on medium speed until creamy. Beat in vanilla.

2. Add flour mixed with baking powder and salt and beat until blended. Stir in chocolate chips and nuts.

3. Shape dough into 1-inch balls and place 1½ inches apart on ungreased foil- or parchment-lined cookie sheets. Press each gently to flatten. Bake 35 to 40 minutes, until golden. Remove to a rack and let cool completely.

155 TROPICAL TREASURES

Prep: 10 minutes   Bake: 10 to 12 minutes   Makes: about 44

½ cup solid vegetable shortening	¼ teaspoon baking soda
2 tablespoons butter, softened	¼ teaspoon salt
½ cup granulated sugar	½ cup flaked coconut
¼ cup firmly packed brown sugar	½ cup semisweet chocolate chips
1 egg	¼ cup coarsely chopped dried pineapple
½ teaspoon vanilla extract	¼ cup coarsely chopped raw cashews
1 cup flour	

1. Preheat oven to 350°F. In a large bowl, beat shortening, butter, granulated sugar, and brown sugar with an electric mixer on medium speed until well blended. Beat in egg and vanilla until light and fluffy.

2. Add flour mixed with baking soda and salt and beat until dough is smooth, scraping down side of bowl frequently with a rubber spatula. Fold in coconut, chocolate chips, pineapple, and cashews.

3. Drop by heaping teaspoonfuls 2 inches apart onto lightly greased cookie sheets. Bake 10 to 12 minutes, or until edges are golden brown. To keep cookies chewy, centers should look pale. Let cookies cool 2 minutes on sheets, then remove to racks and let cool completely. Store in a tightly covered container.

Chapter 6

Chocolatey Brownies

Brownies, quite simply, were named for their rich, dark, chocolatey color. And although chocolate has been paired with sugar in sweet pastries for over 300 years (it was first introduced to Europe from America in the early sixteenth century), brownies have only been a part of our sweet tooth since the late 1890s. At first considered a very rich and crusty cake, they have now joined the cookie family as an especially deep, soft-centered bar cookie. Brownies are often divided into cakelike and fudgelike categories. In this chapter, we have a variety of each, with an assortment of toppings and add-ins.

When asked to describe the ideal brownie, "decadent" is the word that most people think of first. When asked to describe "decadent," the range of descriptors widens greatly. While some people want gooey, deep chocolate chunks, others seek mile-high, mild chocolate wedges, full of nuts, raisins, and chocolate chips. Some prefer chewy, while others like cakey. We know some people who have devoted years to the quest for their ideal brownie. As we searched for a collection of sumptuous brownies to suit many tastes, we hoped that many of you would find your perfect brownie in these pages.

Because of the different natures of various brownies, it is sometimes difficult to tell you how to know when brownies are done. The usual tests for cakes and cookies are not always accurate for soft-centered brownies, and brownies don't always pull away from the sides of the pan until they are overdone. We have tried to give you a way of telling when each brownie is perfectly baked, but you will find that the descriptions vary with the kind of brownie. When we note that a brownie is done when a toothpick inserted in the center comes out with a few moist crumbs clinging to it, it is probably because we tried to bake them until the toothpick came out clean and ate a pan of overbaked brownies. Although we really didn't complain about having to try again and eat the pan of perfectly baked brownies, we want all of yours to be perfect.

Because of their variety, it is especially important to bake brownies in the proper size pans and at the exact oven temperature. With all cookie and brownie baking, it is important to keep an oven thermometer in your oven to make sure it is accurate. And no matter which of our recipes you use, the baking time is dependent upon the cookies or brownies going into an oven that has been preheated to the right temperature.

156   BAKING PAN BROWNIES
Prep: 5 minutes   Bake: 22 to 25 minutes   Makes: 16

Because these cakelike brownies are mixed in the baking pan, you can whip up a batch in no time.

¾ cup sugar
¾ cup flour
½ cup chopped walnuts
¼ cup unsweetened cocoa
    powder

1 teaspoon baking powder
¼ teaspoon salt
½ cup water
¼ cup vegetable oil
1 teaspoon vanilla extract

1. Preheat oven to 350°F. Generously grease a 9-inch square pan.

2. In greased pan, with a fork, stir together sugar, flour, walnuts, cocoa, baking powder, and salt until well blended.

3. Add water, oil, and vanilla; stir with fork until uniformly combined.

4. Bake 22 to 25 minutes, or until a toothpick inserted in center comes out clean. Remove pan to a rack, cut into 16 squares, and let cool completely. Brownies have a tendency to stick, so store in pan, tightly wrapped, and serve directly from pan.

157   CARAMEL CHOCOLATE BROWNIES
Prep: 15 minutes   Bake: 25 to 30 minutes   Makes: 36

These irresistible fudgy brownies have melted caramel streaked through them.

1½ sticks (6 ounces) butter,
    melted
¾ cup unsweetened cocoa
    powder
¾ cup granulated sugar
½ cup firmly packed dark
    brown sugar
2 eggs

1 teaspoon vanilla extract
¾ cup flour
¼ teaspoon salt
⅔ cup semisweet chocolate
    chips
20 soft caramel squares (about
    5½ ounces)

1. Preheat oven to 350°F. In a medium bowl, stir together melted butter and cocoa powder until well blended and smooth. Mix in granulated sugar and brown sugar. Beat in eggs and vanilla until well blended.

2. Add flour and salt and beat until blended. Stir in chocolate chips. Turn dough into a greased 8-inch square pan, leveling surface.

3. In a microwave-safe bowl, combine caramels with 2 tablespoons water. Microwave at 50 percent power for 2 to 3 minutes, stirring occasionally, until caramels melt. Drizzle caramel over dough in pan and swirl through, using a knife.

4. Bake 25 to 30 minutes, or until edges are set. Remove pan to a rack and let cool completely before cutting into 36 squares.

158   BLACKOUT BROWNIES
Prep: 20 minutes   Bake: 12 to 15 minutes   Makes: 16

For those times when nothing but chocolate will do, these dark chocolate brownies are a chocolate lover's dream come true.

1 stick (4 ounces) butter	1 cup flour
3 (1-ounce) squares unsweetened chocolate	½ teaspoon baking powder
	¼ teaspoon salt
1 cup sugar	3 (1-ounce) squares semisweet chocolate
2 eggs	
2 teaspoons vanilla extract	¼ cup heavy cream

1. Preheat oven to 350°F. Grease an 8-inch square pan and a 6-inch round in center of a cookie sheet.

2. In a medium saucepan, melt butter and unsweetened chocolate over low heat, stirring until smooth. Remove from heat, turn into a medium bowl, and set aside 10 minutes to cool slightly.

3. With an electric mixer on medium speed, beat sugar, eggs, and vanilla into cooled chocolate mixture. Mix together flour, baking powder, and salt and fold in to make a thick batter. Remove ¼ cup batter; spread onto greased round on cookie sheet. Turn remaining batter into prepared pan, leveling surface.

4. Place both brownie pans in oven. Bake brownie round 5 to 6 minutes, or until crisp. Bake pan of brownies 12 to 15 minutes, or until a toothpick inserted in center comes out clean. Slide brownie round onto a wire rack and let cool completely. Set square brownie in pan on a rack to cool.

5. Meanwhile, chop semisweet chocolate. In a small saucepan, heat chocolate and cream over low heat, stirring until smooth. Or combine chocolate and cream in a glass measuring cup and microwave on High 1 to 1½ minutes, or until chocolate is melted; stir until smooth. Pour over baked brownie in square pan.

6. Break brownie round from cookie sheet into pieces. Place pieces in a plastic bag and roll to make crumbs. Sprinkle brownie crumbs over frosted brownie in pan. Cut into 16 squares and let cool completely. Store in an airtight container or wrap well and refrigerate.

159 CHOCOLATE CHEWS
Prep: 10 minutes   Bake: 20 to 25 minutes   Makes: 16

When baked, the marshmallows melt, making these brownies extra chewy.

½ cup flour
½ teaspoon baking powder
⅛ teaspoon salt
1 stick (4 ounces) butter, melted
½ cup unsweetened cocoa powder

1 cup sugar
2 eggs
1 teaspoon vanilla extract
½ cup mini marshmallows
½ cup semisweet chocolate chips

1. Preheat oven to 350°F. Grease an 8-inch square pan. In a small bowl, combine flour, baking powder, and salt.

2. In a medium bowl, stir together melted butter and cocoa powder until blended. Stir in sugar, then add eggs, one at a time, beating well after each addition. Stir in vanilla.

3. Add flour mixture and mix until well blended. Stir in marshmallows and chocolate chips.

4. Turn batter into prepared pan, leveling surface with a rubber scraper. Bake 20 to 25 minutes, until a toothpick inserted in center comes out with a few moist crumbs clinging to it. Remove pan to a rack. Let cool completely in pan before cutting into 16 squares.

160 CHOCOLATE ALMOND DECADENCE
Prep: 20 minutes   Bake: 25 to 30 minutes   Makes: 16

¾ cup flour
½ teaspoon baking powder
Pinch of salt
1½ sticks (6 ounces) butter
½ cup unsweetened cocoa powder

1 cup sugar
2 eggs
1 teaspoon almond extract
½ teaspoon vanilla extract
7 ounces almond paste

1. Preheat oven to 350°F. Grease an 8-inch square baking pan. Combine flour, baking powder, and salt.

2. Melt butter over low heat or in a microwave. In a medium bowl, combine melted butter and cocoa powder; stir until well blended. Mix in sugar. Add eggs, one at a time, beating well after each addition. Stir in almond extract and vanilla. Stir in flour mixture until blended. Spread half of batter into bottom of prepared pan.

3. Roll almond paste into an 8-inch square. Place on top of batter in pan. Top with remaining batter. Bake 25 to 30 minutes, until edges begin to pull away from sides of pan. Remove pan to a rack. Let cool completely in pan before cutting into 16 squares.

161 CHUNKY CHOCOLATE BROWNIES
Prep: 7 minutes   Bake: 25 to 30 minutes   Makes: 16

1 stick (4 ounces) butter,
   softened
1 cup firmly packed brown
   sugar
3 (1-ounce) squares
   unsweetened chocolate,
   melted

1 teaspoon vanilla extract
2 eggs
⅔ cup flour
¼ teaspoon salt
6 ounces semisweet chocolate
   chunks (1 cup)
½ cup chopped pecans

1. Preheat oven to 350°F. Grease a 9-inch square pan.

2. In a medium bowl, beat butter, brown sugar, melted chocolate, and vanilla with an electric mixer on medium speed until smooth. Add eggs, one at a time, beating well after each addition. Add flour and salt and beat on low speed just until batter is smooth, scraping side of bowl frequently with a rubber spatula. Fold in chocolate chunks and nuts. Turn batter into prepared pan, leveling surface.

3. Bake 25 to 30 minutes, or until top is shiny and dry and a toothpick inserted in center comes out clean. Remove pan to a rack, cut into 16 squares, and let cool completely. Store in an airtight container.

162 CHOCOLATE CHUNK FUDGY BROWNIES
Prep: 7 minutes   Bake: 20 to 25 minutes   Makes: 24

These fudgy brownies are Bonnie's favorite. The recipe takes only about 7 minutes to prepare, so it's great when you're in a rush.

2 sticks (8 ounces) butter
¾ cup unsweetened cocoa
   powder
2 cups sugar
4 eggs, at room temperature
2 teaspoons vanilla extract

1 cup flour
½ teaspoon salt
12 ounces semisweet chocolate
   chunks (2 cups)
1 cup chopped nuts (optional)

1. Preheat oven to 350°F. Grease a 13 × 9 × 2-inch baking pan.

2. Melt butter over low heat or in a microwave. Scrape into a medium bowl. Add cocoa powder and stir until well blended. Mix in sugar. Add eggs, one at a time, beating well after each addition. Stir in vanilla, then flour and salt. Do not overbeat. Stir in chocolate chunks and, if desired, nuts.

3. Turn into prepared pan, leveling surface. Bake 20 to 25 minutes, or until a toothpick inserted near center comes out with just a few moist crumbs clinging to it. Remove pan to a rack. Let cool completely in pan before cutting into 24 bars.

Recipe reprinted courtesy of *Saco Foods*.

163   FROSTED FUDGY COCOA BROWNIES
Prep: 10 minutes   Bake: 20 to 25 minutes   Makes: 16

1 stick (4 ounces) plus
   2½ tablespoons butter
⅓ cup plus 2½ tablespoons
   unsweetened cocoa
   powder
1 cup granulated sugar
2 eggs

1¾ teaspoons vanilla extract
½ cup flour
¼ teaspoon salt
½ cup chopped pecans
1 cup powdered sugar
1 tablespoon milk

1. Preheat oven to 350°F. Melt 1 stick butter over low heat or in a microwave. Scrape into a medium bowl. Add ⅓ cup cocoa powder and stir until well blended.

2. Add sugar and mix well. Add eggs, one at a time, beating well after each addition. Beat in 1 teaspoon vanilla, then flour and salt. Do not overbeat. Stir in pecans.

3. Turn into a greased 8-inch square pan, leveling surface. Bake 20 to 25 minutes, or until a toothpick inserted near center comes out with a few moist crumbs clinging to it. Remove pan to a rack and let cool completely.

4. Melt 2½ tablespoons butter over low heat or in a microwave. Scrape into a medium bowl, add remaining 2½ tablespoons cocoa powder, and stir until well blended. Mix in remaining ¾ teaspoon vanilla. With an electric mixer on medium speed, beat in powdered sugar and milk until smooth, fluffy, and of spreading consistency. Spread on cooled brownies, then cut into 16 squares.

Recipe reprinted courtesy of *Saco Foods*.

164   BUTTERMILK BROWNIES
Prep: 15 minutes   Bake: 18 to 20 minutes   Makes: 50

Our friend Amy Barr, *Good Housekeeping* Institute's director, shared these luscious fudge-topped bars with us.

2 cups granulated sugar
2 cups flour
½ cup plus 2 tablespoons
   unsweetened cocoa
   powder
3 tablespoons buttermilk
   powder
1 teaspoon baking soda

½ teaspoon salt
2 sticks (8 ounces) plus 6
   tablespoons butter
½ cup vegetable oil
2 eggs
1 tablespoon vanilla extract
1½ cups chopped walnuts
4 cups powdered sugar

1. Preheat oven to 350°F. Grease and flour a 10 × 15 × 1-inch jelly-roll pan. In a large bowl, stir together granulated sugar, flour, ¼ cup cocoa powder, buttermilk powder, baking soda, and ¼ teaspoon salt.

2. In a medium saucepan, combine 2 sticks butter, oil, and 1½ cups water. Bring to a boil over medium heat. Pour hot liquid over sugar-flour mixture and stir until well blended. Beat in eggs and 1 teaspoon vanilla. Stir in 1 cup walnuts.

3. Pour into prepared jelly-roll pan and level surface. Bake 18 to 20 minutes, or until a toothpick inserted in center comes out with a few crumbs clinging to it. Remove pan to a rack to cool.

4. In a medium bowl, combine powdered sugar with remaining ¼ cup plus 2 tablespoons cocoa powder, 6 tablespoons softened butter, 2 teaspoons vanilla, and ¼ teaspoon salt. Add ⅓ cup water and beat with an electric mixer on medium speed until blended. Add up to 3 tablespoons more water to make a spreadable frosting.

5. Spread over cooled brownies, sprinkle remaining ½ cup walnuts on top, and cut into 50 bars.

---

165 AMARETTI BROWNIES
Prep: 15 minutes   Bake: 20 to 25 minutes   Makes: 16

These almond-infused brownies are for that extra special occasion. They take a bit more time to make than some of our others, but we think they are well worth the effort.

5 (1-ounce) squares semisweet chocolate	¾ cup firmly packed dark brown sugar
12 double amaretti biscuits, crumbled (⅔ cup crumbs)	1 stick (4 ounces) plus 2 tablespoons butter, softened
½ cup toasted chopped almonds	3 eggs
⅓ cup flour	1 teaspoon almond extract

1. Preheat oven to 350°F. Grease a 9-inch square pan. Melt chocolate over low heat in a double boiler set over simmering water or in a microwave. Remove from heat and set aside.

2. In a food processor, finely grind amaretti biscuits and almonds. Mix in flour. Remove and set aside.

3. In a large bowl, blend brown sugar and butter until creamy. Add eggs, one at a time, beating well after each addition. Stir in melted chocolate and almond extract. Mix in almond-flour mixture just until combined.

4. Turn into prepared pan, leveling surface. Bake 20 to 25 minutes, until a toothpick inserted in center comes out with a few moist crumbs clinging to it. Remove pan to a rack and let cool completely in pan before cutting into 16 squares.

166   COCONUT BROWNIES
Prep: 7 minutes   Bake: 20 to 25 minutes   Makes: 16

6 tablespoons butter	1 teaspoon vanilla extract
2 (1-ounce) squares unsweetened chocolate	⅔ cup cake flour
	½ teaspoon baking powder
1 cup sugar	¼ teaspoon salt
2 eggs	¾ cup flaked coconut

1. Preheat oven to 350°F. In a small heatproof bowl in a microwave oven on High power or in a double boiler over hot water, melt butter and chocolate, Stir until smooth and well blended.

2. In a medium bowl, beat sugar into chocolate butter, until well blended. Add eggs, one at a time, beating well after each addition. Stir in vanilla, then cake flour mixed with baking powder and salt. Stir in coconut. Turn into a greased 8-inch square pan, leveling surface.

3. Bake 20 to 25 minutes, or until a toothpick inserted near center comes out with a few moist crumbs clinging to it. Remove pan to a rack. Let cool completely in pan before cutting into 16 squares.

167   FRUIT AND CREAM CHEESE BROWNIES
*Prep: 15 minutes   Stand: 2 to 3 hours   Bake: 30 to 35 minutes
Makes: 16*

Tart chewy dried fruit, creamy sweet cheesecake, and dense chocolatey brownie make these a study in contrasts.

2 tablespoons chopped dried sour cherries	1 stick (4 ounces) butter, softened
2 tablespoons chopped dried apricots	⅓ cup sugar
	2 eggs
2 tablespoons chopped raisins	2 teaspoons vanilla extract
¼ cup Cointreau or other orange-flavored liqueur	2 (1-ounce) squares unsweetened chocolate, melted
⅓ cup flour	8 ounces cream cheese, softened
¼ teaspoon baking powder	
¼ teaspoon salt	

1. In a small bowl, combine cherries, apricots, raisins, and Cointreau. Let stand at room temperature 2 to 3 hours.

2. Preheat oven to 350°F. Grease a 9-inch square pan. In a small bowl, stir together flour, baking powder, and salt.

3. In a large bowl, beat butter and sugar with an electric mixer on medium speed until fluffy. Beat in 1 egg and vanilla until smooth. Add flour mixture; beat on low speed until a smooth, stiff batter forms, scraping down side of bowl frequently with a rubber spatula.

4. Stir melted chocolate into batter. Remove and reserve ¼ cup chocolate batter. Turn remaining chocolate batter into prepared pan, leveling surface.

5. Add cream cheese and remaining egg to fruit mixture and stir with a fork until well blended. Spoon fruit mixture on top of chocolate batter in pan. Drizzle reserved chocolate batter over top.

6. Bake 30 to 35 minutes, or until center is set and top is lightly browned. Remove pan to a rack, cut into 16 squares, and let cool completely. Store, covered, in refrigerator.

---

168 GERMAN CHOCOLATE BROWNIES
Prep: 10 minutes   Bake: 20 to 25 minutes   Makes: 16

1 stick (4 ounces) butter
4 ounces sweet baking chocolate
⅓ cup flour
1 teaspoon cinnamon
½ teaspoon baking powder
¼ teaspoon salt
2 eggs

½ cup granulated sugar
1 teaspoon vanilla extract
⅓ cup firmly packed brown sugar
⅓ cup heavy cream
⅓ cup chopped pecans
⅓ cup flaked coconut

1. Preheat oven to 350°F. In a small saucepan over very low heat or in a microwave, melt ½ stick (4 tablespoons) butter and chocolate together; set aside to cool to room temperature. Grease a 9-inch square pan. In a medium bowl, stir together flour, cinnamon, baking powder, and salt.

2. In a large bowl, with an electric mixer on high speed, beat eggs until thick and lemon colored. Gradually beat in granulated sugar and vanilla.

3. With a wire whisk, fold in melted chocolate mixture and flour mixture until batter is well blended, scraping down side of bowl frequently with a rubber spatula. Turn batter into prepared pan, leveling surface.

4. Bake 20 to 25 minutes, or until center is firm and a toothpick inserted in center comes out clean. Remove pan to a rack and let cool 30 minutes.

5. When brownies have cooled, in a small saucepan, bring remaining ½ stick butter, brown sugar, and cream to a boil. Reduce heat to medium-low and cook, stirring, until slightly thickened, 2 to 3 minutes. Stir in pecans and coconut. Spread topping over brownie layer in pan. Cut into 16 squares and serve warm; or cool, wrap well, and refrigerate.

169 GRAND MARNIER BROWNIES
Prep: 10 minutes   Bake: 25 to 30 minutes   Makes: 16

These chewy brownies have just a hint of orange.

1½ sticks (6 ounces) butter,
   melted
¾ cup unsweetened cocoa
   powder
2 eggs
1½ cups sugar

2 tablespoons Grand Marnier
   or other orange liqueur
½ cup flour
¼ teaspoon salt
2 teaspoons grated orange zest

1. Preheat oven to 350°F. In a small bowl, stir together melted butter and cocoa powder until blended and smooth.

2. In a medium bowl, beat eggs with an electric mixer on medium speed until foamy. Gradually add sugar, beating until light and fluffy. Beat in chocolate butter and Grand Marnier. Stir in flour, salt, and orange zest.

3. Turn batter into a greased 9-inch square pan, leveling surface with a rubber spatula. Bake 25 to 30 minutes, until a toothpick inserted in center comes out with a few moist crumbs clinging to it. Remove pan to a rack and let cool completely in pan before cutting into 16 squares.

170 CHOCOLATE MINT MANIA BARS
Prep: 10 minutes   Bake: 22 to 27 minutes   Makes: 32

4 (1-ounce) squares
   unsweetened chocolate
1½ sticks (6 ounces) butter
2 cups sugar
4 eggs
2 teaspoons vanilla extract
½ teaspoon peppermint extract

1 cup flour
1 teaspoon baking powder
½ teaspoon salt
12 ounces semisweet mint
   chocolate chips (2 cups)
½ cup finely chopped walnuts

1. Preheat oven to 350°F. In a medium bowl in a microwave, melt chocolate and butter on High 2 to 3 minutes, stirring until smooth and blended. Or melt in a small saucepan over low heat.

2. In a medium bowl, mix sugar into chocolate butter. Add eggs, one at a time, beating well after each addition. Stir in vanilla and peppermint extract.

3. Add flour mixed with baking powder and salt. Stir in 1 cup mint chocolate chips. Turn batter into a greased 9 × 13-inch baking pan, leveling surface. Bake 20 to 25 minutes, until a toothpick inserted in center comes out with a few moist crumbs clinging to it.

4. Remove pan from oven, sprinkle remaining 1 cup mint chocolate chips over top, and return to oven for 2 minutes. Remove pan to a wire rack, spread chips over top, and sprinkle with walnuts. Let cool completely in pan before cutting into 32 bars.

171 CHOCOLATE AFTER-DINNER MINT SQUARES

Prep: 15 minutes   Bake: 10 to 15 minutes   Makes: 36

Serve these bar cookies as you would after-dinner mint candies.

3 (1-ounce) squares unsweetened chocolate	6 tablespoons flour Pinch of salt
6 tablespoons butter	½ cup powdered sugar
1 egg	1 tablespoon crème de menthe
¾ cup granulated sugar	¼ cup semisweet chocolate
¼ teaspoon peppermint extract	chips, melted

1. Preheat oven to 350°F. In a glass bowl in a microwave oven on High or in a double boiler over hot water, melt chocolate and butter, stirring until smooth and blended.

2. In a medium bowl, beat egg with an electric mixer on medium speed until frothy. Beat in granulated sugar and peppermint extract. Beat in chocolate butter until blended. Mix in flour and salt. Turn into a greased 8-inch square pan, leveling surface.

3. Bake 10 to 15 minutes, until cake tester inserted in center comes out clean. Remove to a rack to cool 5 minutes.

4. In a small bowl, stir together powdered sugar and crème de menthe until of spreading consistency. Spread over cooled base, then drizzle with melted chocolate. Let cool completely before cutting into 36 squares.

172 RICH CHOCOLATE BROWNIES

Prep: 10 minutes   Bake: 20 to 25 minutes   Makes: 16

½ cup flour	5½ tablespoons butter
½ teaspoon baking powder	1 cup sugar
⅛ teaspoon salt	2 eggs
2½ (1-ounce) squares unsweetened chocolate	1 teaspoon vanilla extract
	¾ cup chopped walnuts

1. Preheat oven to 350°F. Grease an 8-inch square pan. In a small bowl, combine flour, baking powder, and salt. Stir to mix well.

2. Melt chocolate and butter over low heat in a double boiler set over simmering water or in a microwave. Scrape melted chocolate and butter into a medium bowl. Stir in sugar, then add eggs, one at a time, beating well after each addition. Blend in vanilla. Add flour mixture and beat until blended.

3. Turn batter into prepared pan, leveling surface with a rubber scraper. Sprinkle walnuts over top. Bake 20 to 25 minutes, until a toothpick inserted in center comes out with a few moist crumbs clinging to it. Remove pan to a rack and let cool completely in pan before cutting into 16 squares.

173 MOCHA BROWNIES
Prep: 10 minutes   Bake: 20 to 25 minutes   Makes: 20

These brownies are even better the second day, as the coffee flavor intensifies with storage.

½ cup flour
2 tablespoons finely ground French roast or espresso coffee
¼ teaspoon salt
1 stick (4 ounces) butter, softened

¾ cup sugar
3 eggs
3 (1-ounce) squares unsweetened chocolate, melted
2 tablespoons coffee-flavored liqueur

1. Preheat oven to 350°F. Grease a 9-inch square pan. In a medium bowl, stir together flour, coffee, and salt.

2. In a large bowl, beat butter and sugar with an electric mixer on medium speed until fluffy. Beat in eggs, one at a time, until very fluffy. Beat in melted chocolate and liqueur.

3. Add flour mixture to sugar mixture. Beat on low speed until batter is smooth, scraping down side of bowl frequently with a rubber spatula. Turn batter into prepared pan, leveling surface.

4. Bake brownies 20 to 25 minutes, or until surface is dry and a toothpick inserted in center comes out with a few moist crumbs clinging to it. Remove pan to a rack, cut into 20 rectangles, and let cool completely. Store in an airtight container or wrap well and refrigerate.

174 PRUNE BROWNIES
Prep: 15 minutes   Bake: 20 to 25 minutes   Makes: 16

Surprisingly, the substitution of prune puree for the butter in this recipe produces a moist, chocolatey brownie which, if you use the egg whites and omit the optional walnuts, is very low in fat.

⅔ cup pitted prunes
¾ cup flour
½ cup sugar
⅓ cup unsweetened cocoa powder
½ teaspoon baking powder

¼ teaspoon salt
2 whole eggs or 4 egg whites
2 teaspoons vanilla extract
½ cup chopped walnuts (optional)

1. In a food processor, puree prunes until smooth. Set prune puree aside.

2. Preheat oven to 350°F. Grease an 8-inch square pan. In a medium bowl, stir together flour, sugar, cocoa powder, baking powder, and salt.

3. Add prune puree, eggs, and vanilla; beat on low speed just until a stiff batter forms, scraping down side of bowl frequently with a rubber spatula. Fold in nuts, if desired. Turn batter into prepared pan, leveling surface.

4. Bake 20 to 25 minutes, or until top looks dry and a toothpick inserted in center comes out clean. Remove pan to a rack, cut into 16 squares, and let cool completely. Store in an airtight container or wrap well and refrigerate.

---

175 OATMEAL-RAISIN BROWNIES
Prep: 15 minutes   Bake: 20 to 25 minutes   Makes: 20

We discovered these one day when we had only half the flour needed to bake brownies and we've been making them ever since.

1 stick (4 ounces) butter	1 cup flour
3 (1-ounce) squares	1 cup rolled oats
unsweetened chocolate	½ teaspoon baking powder
1 cup sugar	¼ teaspoon salt
2 eggs	½ cup raisins
2 teaspoons vanilla extract	

1. Preheat oven to 350°F. Grease a 9-inch square pan.

2. In a medium saucepan, melt butter and chocolate over low heat, stirring until smooth. Remove from heat, turn into a medium bowl, and set aside 10 minutes to cool slightly.

3. With an electric mixer set on medium speed, beat sugar, eggs, and vanilla into cooled chocolate mixture. Fold in flour mixed with oatmeal, baking powder, and salt to make a thick batter. Fold in raisins. Turn into prepared pan, leveling surface.

4. Bake 20 to 25 minutes, or until a toothpick inserted in center comes out clean. Remove pan to a rack, cut into 20 rectangles, and let cool completely. Store in an airtight container or wrap well and refrigerate.

176   ROCKY ROAD BROWNIES
Prep: 10 minutes   Bake: 20 to 22 minutes   Makes: 16

½ cup sugar
1 stick (4 ounces) butter, softened
1 teaspoon vanilla extract
½ cup flour
2 tablespoons unsweetened cocoa powder

¼ teaspoon salt
½ cup coarsely chopped hazelnuts
6 ounces white baking chips (1 cup)
6 ounces semisweet chocolate chips (1 cup)

1. Preheat oven to 350°F. Grease an 8-inch square pan.

2. In a small bowl, beat sugar, butter, and vanilla with an electric mixer on medium speed until fluffy. At low speed, beat in flour, cocoa powder, and salt until a stiff batter forms, scraping down side of bowl frequently with a rubber spatula. Turn half of batter into prepared pan. With rubber spatula, spread to make an even layer.

3. Sprinkle hazelnuts and white and chocolate chips over dough. Drop remaining batter by teaspoonfuls over chips.

4. Bake 20 to 22 minutes, or until surface is dry and a toothpick inserted in center comes out with a few moist crumbs clinging to it. Remove pan to a rack, cut into 16 squares, and let cool completely. Store in an airtight container.

177   POLKA DOT SQUARES
Prep: 10 minutes   Bake: 20 to 25 minutes   Makes: 16

This is a classic blond brownie, studded with dots of chocolate. If your family likes nuts, add about ½ cup along with the chocolate chips.

1 cup flour
½ teaspoon baking powder
¼ teaspoon salt
6 tablespoons butter, softened
1 cup firmly packed dark brown sugar

1 egg
1 teaspoon vanilla extract
6 ounces semisweet chocolate chips (1 cup)

1. Preheat oven to 350°F. Grease an 8-inch square pan. In a small bowl, combine flour, baking powder, and salt.

2. In a large bowl, beat butter and brown sugar until fluffy. Beat in egg and vanilla with an electric mixer on medium speed until smooth. Add flour mixture and beat on low speed until batter is smooth, scraping down side of bowl frequently with a rubber spatula. Stir in chocolate chips. Turn into prepared pan, leveling surface.

3. Bake 20 to 25 minutes, until a toothpick inserted in center comes out with a few moist crumbs clinging to it. Remove pan to a rack. Let cool completely in pan before cutting into 16 squares.

178 PEANUT BUTTER BROWNIE SANDWICHES
Prep: 15 minutes   Bake: 15 to 18 minutes   Makes: 16

1 cup flour
1 teaspoon baking powder
¼ teaspoon salt
¾ cup sugar
1 stick (4 ounces) butter, softened
2 eggs
¼ cup dark corn syrup
2 (1-ounce) squares unsweetened chocolate, melted
1 teaspoon vanilla extract
½ cup chunky peanut butter

1. Preheat oven to 350°F. Generously grease a 13 × 9-inch baking pan. In a medium bowl, stir together flour, baking powder, and salt.

2. In a large bowl, beat sugar, butter, eggs, corn syrup, melted chocolate, and vanilla with an electric mixer on medium speed until smooth. Add flour mixture; beat on low speed just until batter is smooth, scraping down side of bowl frequently with a rubber spatula. Turn batter into prepared pan, leveling surface.

3. Bake 15 to 18 minutes, or until top is firm and a toothpick inserted in center comes out clean. Remove pan to a wire rack; let cool 15 minutes in pan on rack. Loosen edges of brownie; invert onto rack and let cool completely.

4. Cut cooled brownie in half crosswise. Spread one half with peanut butter. Top with other half of brownie. Cut into 16 bars and store in an airtight container.

179 CHOCOLATE ROCKY ROAD BARS
Prep: 10 minutes   Bake: 28 to 34 minutes   Makes: 20

6 tablespoons butter, melted
6 tablespoons unsweetened cocoa powder
1 cup sugar
2 eggs
⅔ cup flour
1 teaspoon vanilla extract
¼ teaspoon salt
1½ cups miniature marshmallows
¾ cup semisweet chocolate chips
½ cup chopped salted peanuts

1. Preheat oven to 350°F. In a medium bowl, combine melted butter and cocoa powder. Stir until well blended. Mix in sugar. Add eggs, one at a time, beating well after each addition. Stir in flour, vanilla, and salt.

2. Turn into a greased 9-inch square pan, leveling surface. Bake 18 to 22 minutes, until brownies begin to pull away from sides of pan. Remove from oven; leave oven on.

3. Sprinkle marshmallows, chocolate chips, and peanuts over brownies. Return to oven and bake 10 to 12 minutes, until marshmallows are lightly browned. Remove to a rack and let cool completely before cutting into 20 bars.

180 TRIPLE CHOCOLATE BROWNIES
Prep: 10 minutes   Bake: 20 to 25 minutes   Makes: 20

¾ cup flour
6 tablespoons unsweetened cocoa powder
½ teaspoon baking powder
¼ teaspoon salt
1¼ sticks (6 ounces) butter, softened

1 cup sugar
2 eggs
1 teaspoon vanilla extract
½ cup white baking chips
½ cup semisweet chocolate chips

1. Preheat oven to 350°F. Grease an 8-inch square pan. In a small bowl, stir together flour, cocoa powder, baking powder, and salt.

2. In a large bowl, beat butter with an electric mixer on medium speed until creamy. Gradually beat in sugar until fluffy. Add eggs, one at a time, beating well after each addition. Beat in vanilla.

3. Add flour mixture and beat on low speed until batter is smooth, scraping down side of bowl frequently with a rubber spatula. Stir in white and semisweet chocolate chips. Turn batter into prepared pan, leveling surface.

4. Bake 20 to 25 minutes, until a toothpick inserted in center comes out with a few moist crumbs clinging to it. Remove to a rack. Let cool completely in pan before cutting into 20 bars.

181 TUXEDO BARS
Prep: 10 minutes   Bake: 28 to 34 minutes   Makes: 20

1 stick (4 ounces) butter, softened
2 (1-ounce) squares semisweet chocolate, melted
⅓ cup unsweetened cocoa powder
1½ cups sugar
4 eggs

1 teaspoon vanilla extract
1 cup flour
¼ teaspoon salt
2 cups miniature marshmallows
1 (1-ounce) square unsweetened chocolate, melted

1. Preheat oven to 350°F. In a medium bowl, beat butter, melted semisweet chocolate, cocoa powder, sugar, eggs, and vanilla with an electric mixer on medium speed until smooth.

2. Add flour and salt. Beat on low speed just until batter is smooth, scraping down side of bowl frequently with a rubber spatula. Turn batter into a greased 9-inch square pan, leveling surface.

3. Bake 25 to 30 minutes, or until a toothpick inserted near center comes out with a few moist crumbs clinging to it. Sprinkle marshmallows evenly over baked brownies and return to oven for 3 to 4 minutes to soften marshmallows.

4. Remove pan to a rack. Drizzle melted unsweetened chocolate decoratively over marshmallows. Let cool completely before cutting into 20 bars.

Chapter 7

Golden Brownies

Now, we all know that there is no such thing as a golden brownie, because brownies got their name from their rich brown color, and if it isn't chocolate brown it isn't a brownie. But there is also no such thing as the ideal name for a golden bar cookie with the same variety of textures and temperaments as its rich chocolatey cousin. Should we call them light brownies, golden bars, blondies? Whatever, in this chapter we explore the lighter side of the brownie question, with a selection of sweet, seductive squares and bars, some dense and gooey, some high and stuffed with hidden treasures.

Brownies, both dark and light, are best when eaten the day they are baked. Although some store better than others, most tend to dry out quickly once several pieces have been removed from the pan. To keep them moist as long as possible, brownies should be cooled completely on a wire rack and then wrapped in plastic wrap or slipped into a plastic bag while still in their baking pan.

Although they may dry out quickly at room temperature, brownies and golden brownies, or blondies, freeze very well. You can bake, cool, and wrap whole pans of them for later use; or once cool, you can wrap individual pieces and freeze them in a plastic bag or freezer container and remove them individually as needed. Individually frozen brownies can be popped into a lunch bag and, in addition to keeping other foods cool, they thaw to moist perfection by lunchtime. A few frozen brownies can be unwrapped and warmed in the oven or microwave while you are making a pot of coffee for unexpected guests.

182 BURNT-SUGAR BLONDIES
Prep: 15 minutes   Bake: 20 to 25 minutes   Makes: 16

Caramelized sugar syrup adds both flavor and moisture to these golden squares.

1 cup sugar	¼ teaspoon salt
½ cup boiling water	6 tablespoons butter, softened
½ teaspoon lemon juice	1 egg
1 cup flour	2 teaspoons vanilla extract
¼ teaspoon baking powder	1 cup chopped walnuts

1. In a small saucepan, combine sugar, ¼ cup boiling water, and lemon juice. Heat to boiling, stirring to dissolve sugar. Cook over high heat, stirring constantly, until mixture is golden brown. Immediately remove from heat and very carefully stir in remaining ¼ cup boiling water. Pour caramel into a 2-cup glass measuring cup. If necessary, stir in enough cold water to make ⅔ cup. Set aside to cool.

2. Preheat oven to 350°F. Grease a 9-inch square pan. In a medium bowl, stir together flour, baking powder, and salt.

3. In a large bowl, beat butter, egg, and vanilla with an electric mixer on medium speed until smooth. Add flour mixture and ⅔ cup cooled caramel; beat on low speed until batter is smooth, scraping down side of bowl frequently with a rubber spatula.

4. Fold in ¾ cup walnuts. Turn batter into prepared pan, leveling surface. Sprinkle remaining ¼ cup nuts over top.

5. Bake 20 to 25 minutes, or until top is golden brown and a toothpick inserted in center comes out clean. Remove pan to a rack, cut into 16 squares, and let cool completely. Store in an airtight container or wrap well and refrigerate.

183 BROWN-SUGAR BLONDIES
Prep: 15 minutes   Bake: 20 to 25 minutes   Makes: 16

Golden raisins add an additional touch of sweetness to these butterscotchy squares.

1 cup flour	1 stick (4 ounces) butter, softened
¾ teaspoon baking powder	
¼ teaspoon salt	2 eggs
1¾ cups firmly packed brown sugar	2 teaspoons vanilla extract
	½ cup chopped walnuts
	½ cup golden raisins

1. Preheat oven to 350°F. Grease a 9-inch square pan. In a medium bowl, stir together flour, baking powder, and salt.

2. In a large bowl, beat brown sugar and butter with an electric mixer on medium speed until fluffy. Add eggs and vanilla and beat until smooth. Add flour mixture; beat on low speed until batter is smooth, scraping down side of bowl frequently with a rubber spatula. Fold in nuts and golden raisins. Turn batter into prepared pan, leveling surface.

3. Bake 20 to 25 minutes, or until top is golden brown and a toothpick inserted in center comes out clean. Remove pan to a rack, cut into 16 squares, and let cool completely. Store in an airtight container or wrap well and refrigerate.

---

184 FLOURLESS BLOND BROWNIES
Prep: 10 minutes   Bake: 35 to 38 minutes   Makes: 16

Beth Hillson, an author, food journalist, and friend, shared her gluten-free brownie recipe with us. If you didn't know, you couldn't tell it was made without flour. According to Beth, those on a severe gluten restriction diet should purchase gluten-free vanilla.

¾ cup soy flour
¼ cup potato starch
¼ cup cornstarch
¾ teaspoon baking powder
½ teaspoon salt
½ teaspoon xanthan gum
   (optional; see Note)

1 stick (4 ounces) butter, softened
1 cup firmly packed light brown sugar
2 eggs
1 teaspoon vanilla extract
¾ cup toasted pecans
½ cup semisweet chocolate chips

1. Preheat oven to 350°F. Coat a 9-inch square pan with vegetable oil spray.

2. In a small bowl, stir together soy flour, potato starch, cornstarch, baking powder, salt, and xanthan gum, if using.

3. In a medium bowl, beat butter and brown sugar with an electric mixer on medium speed until fluffy. Add eggs and vanilla and beat well. Add dry mixture and stir with a large spoon to combine. Fold in toasted pecans and chocolate chips. Turn into prepared pan, leveling surface.

4. Bake 35 to 38 minutes, until a toothpick inserted in center comes out with a few moist crumbs clinging to it. Remove pan to a rack. Let cool completely in pan before cutting into 16 squares.

   NOTE: *Xanthan gum is available in health food stores.*

185 WHOLE WHEAT BUTTERSCOTCH BROWNIES

Prep: 10 minutes   Bake: 25 to 30 minutes   Makes: 25

Although these blond brownies could be made entirely of white flour, the whole wheat flour gives them added texture and flavor.

1 cup all-purpose flour
1 cup whole wheat flour
2 teaspoons baking powder
¼ teaspoon salt
1 stick (4 ounces) butter, softened

1 cup firmly packed light brown sugar
1 egg
½ cup dark corn syrup
2 teaspoons vanilla extract
1 cup chopped pecans or walnuts

1. Preheat oven to 350°F. Grease a 9 × 13-inch baking pan. In a medium bowl, stir together all-purpose flour, whole wheat flour, baking powder, and salt.

2. In a large bowl, beat butter and brown sugar with an electric mixer on medium speed until fluffy. Beat in egg, corn syrup, and vanilla until smooth.

3. Add flour mixture and beat on low speed until a soft dough forms, scraping down side of bowl frequently with a rubber spatula. Fold ¾ cup nuts into dough. Turn dough into prepared pan, leveling surface. Sprinkle remaining ¼ cup nuts over dough.

4. Bake 25 to 30 minutes, or until top is golden brown and a toothpick inserted in center comes out with a few moist crumbs clinging to it. Remove pan to a rack, cut into 25 bars, and let cool completely. Store in an airtight container or wrap well and refrigerate.

186 HAZELNUT CHEWS

Prep: 20 minutes   Bake: 18 to 20 minutes   Makes: 25

These chewy little blondies are best when eaten freshly baked. To store for a day or two, place them in a tightly closed container with a slice of fresh bread to keep their soft butterscotch centers from drying out.

1½ cups firmly packed brown sugar
1 stick (4 ounces) butter
2 eggs
2 teaspoons vanilla extract
1½ cups flour

1½ teaspoons baking powder
¼ teaspoon salt
1 cup coarsely chopped hazelnuts
½ cup powdered sugar

1. Preheat oven to 350°F. Grease a 9-inch square pan. In a medium saucepan, stir brown sugar and butter over medium-low heat until bubbly; set aside to cool.

2. Add eggs, one at a time, to cooled mixture, beating constantly with a hand-held electric mixer on medium speed until very fluffy. Stir in vanilla.

3. Add flour mixed with baking powder and salt. Beat on low speed until batter is smooth, scraping down side of saucepan frequently with a rubber spatula. Fold in nuts. Turn into prepared pan, leveling surface.

4. Bake 18 to 20 minutes, or until top is set and lightly browned. Do not overbake. Remove pan to a rack, cut into 25 squares, and let cool completely; center will fall as squares cool.

5. Place powdered sugar in a plastic bag. One at a time, drop squares into sugar and shake to coat completely. Store in an airtight container or wrap well and refrigerate.

---

187 CARRARA BROWNIES
Prep: 10 minutes   Bake: 18 to 20 minutes   Makes: 16

This is a simple version of a marbleized brownie. Instead of using both a chocolate and plain batter, melted chocolate chips are swirled through the vanilla batter.

1 **cup flour**	¾ **cup firmly packed dark**
1 **teaspoon baking powder**	**brown sugar**
½ **teaspoon salt**	1 **egg, at room temperature**
1 **stick (4 ounces) butter,**	1 **teaspoon vanilla extract**
softened	6 **ounces semisweet chocolate**
	chips (1 cup)

1. Preheat oven to 350°F. Grease a 9-inch square pan. In a small bowl, stir together flour, baking powder, and salt.

2. In a large bowl, beat butter with an electric mixer on medium speed until creamy. Add brown sugar and beat until fluffy. Beat in egg and vanilla until smooth.

3. Add flour mixture and beat on low speed until dough is smooth, scraping down side of bowl frequently with a rubber spatula. Turn into prepared pan, leveling surface. Sprinkle chocolate chips over batter.

4. Place in oven and bake for 3 minutes, or until chocolate begins to melt. Remove from oven and swirl a knife through dough to marbleize it. Return to oven and bake 15 to 17 minutes longer, until a toothpick inserted in center comes out with a few crumbs clinging to it. Remove pan to a rack. Let cool completely in pan before cutting into 16 squares.

188 PEANUT BUTTER BLONDIES
Prep: 10 minutes   Bake: 20 to 25 minutes   Makes: 32

1¼ cups flour	½ cup chunky peanut butter
1 teaspoon baking powder	2 eggs
¼ teaspoon salt	1½ teaspoons vanilla extract
4 tablespoons butter, softened	½ cup mini chocolate chips
½ cup sugar	(optional)

1. Preheat oven to 350°F. Grease two 8-inch square pans. In a medium bowl, stir together flour, baking powder, and salt.

2. In a large bowl, beat butter, sugar, and peanut butter with an electric mixer on medium speed until blended. Add eggs and vanilla and beat until smooth. Add flour mixture and beat on low speed just until a stiff dough forms, scraping down side of bowl frequently with a rubber spatula. Fold in chocolate chips, if you're adding them. Divide dough between 2 prepared pans, leveling surface.

3. Bake 20 to 25 minutes, or until tops are golden brown and a toothpick inserted in center of each comes out clean. Remove pans to racks, cut each into 16 squares, and let cool completely. Store in a tightly covered container.

189 MRS. STULL'S BLOND BROWNIES
Prep: 10 minutes   Bake: 20 to 25 minutes   Makes: 24

Mrs. Stull, the mother of one of Bonnie's college friends, sent huge cans of these moist golden brownies, studded with chocolate chips, to her daughter Ginger and friends.

1½ sticks (6 ounces) butter, softened	2¼ cups flour
2 cups firmly packed dark brown sugar	1 teaspoon baking powder
	¼ teaspoon salt
2 eggs	6 ounces semisweet chocolate chips (1 cup)
2 teaspoons vanilla extract	

1. Preheat oven to 350°F. Grease a 9 × 13-inch baking pan. In a medium bowl, beat butter and brown sugar with an electric mixer on medium speed until creamy. Beat in eggs and vanilla until well blended.

2. Add flour mixed with baking powder and salt and beat on low speed until blended. Stir in chocolate chips. Turn into prepared pan, leveling surface.

3. Bake 20 to 25 minutes, until a cake tester inserted in center comes out clean. Remove to a rack and let cool completely before cutting into 24 bars.

190 TRADITIONAL BLONDIES
Prep: 15 minutes   Bake: 20 to 25 minutes   Makes: 16

1¼ cups flour
1¼ teaspoons baking powder
¼ teaspoon salt
1 stick (4 ounces) butter,
    softened

1⅓ cups firmly packed brown
    sugar
2 eggs
2 teaspoons vanilla extract
¾ cup chopped pecans or
    walnuts

1. Preheat oven to 350°F. Grease a 9-inch square pan. In a medium bowl, stir together flour, baking powder, and salt.

2. In a large bowl, beat butter and brown sugar with an electric mixer on medium speed until fluffy. Add eggs and vanilla and beat until smooth. Add flour mixture and beat on low speed until thoroughly blended, scraping down side of bowl frequently with a rubber spatula. Fold in nuts. Turn batter into prepared pan, leveling surface.

3. Bake 20 to 25 minutes, or until top is golden brown and a toothpick inserted in center comes out clean. Remove pan to a rack, cut into 16 squares, and let cool completely. Store in an airtight container or wrap well and refrigerate.

---

191 BUTTERSCOTCH TOFFEE BARS
Prep: 10 minutes   Bake: 20 to 25 minutes   Makes: 20

1 stick (4 ounces) butter
1 cup firmly packed brown
    sugar
1 egg

1 teaspoon vanilla extract
¾ cup flour
¼ teaspoon salt
1 cup Heath Bits

1. Preheat oven to 350°F. Grease a 9-inch square pan. Melt butter over low heat or in a microwave. Scrape into a medium bowl. Stir in brown sugar. With an electric mixer on medium speed, beat until well blended, about 2 minutes. Beat in egg, then vanilla.

2. In a small bowl, stir together flour and salt. Add to butter-sugar mixture. Beat on low speed until dough is smooth, scraping down side of bowl frequently with a rubber spatula.

3. Stir in ½ cup Heath Bits. Turn dough into prepared pan, leveling surface. Sprinkle remaining bits over batter.

4. Bake 20 to 25 minutes, or until a toothpick inserted in center comes out with a few moist crumbs clinging to it. Remove pan to a rack. Let cool completely in pan before cutting into 20 bars.

192 COCONUT CONGO BARS
Prep: 10 minutes   Bake: 30 to 35 minutes   Makes: 48

1 stick (4 ounces) plus 5
  tablespoons butter,
  softened
	2½ cups flour

	1 tablespoon baking powder
	1 teaspoon salt

2¼ cups firmly packed dark
  brown sugar
	1½ cups semisweet chocolate
	  chips

3 eggs	1 cup flaked coconut

1. Preheat oven to 350°F. Grease a 9 × 13-inch baking pan. In a medium bowl, beat butter and brown sugar with an electric mixer on medium speed until creamy. Beat in eggs until well blended.

2. Add flour mixed with baking powder and salt and beat until blended. Stir in 1 cup chocolate chips and coconut. Turn into prepared pan, leveling surface.

3. Bake 30 to 35 minutes, until a cake tester inserted in center comes out with a few moist crumbs clinging to it. Remove from oven and immediately sprinkle remaining ½ cup chocolate chips over top. Place on a rack to cool completely before cutting into 48 bars.

193 HONEY WHEAT BLONDIES
Prep: 10 minutes   Bake: 20 to 22 minutes   Makes: 16

½ cup vegetable oil	1 cup whole wheat flour
½ cup honey	1 teaspoon baking powder
½ cup sugar	½ teaspoon baking soda
2 eggs	1 teaspoon cinnamon
1 teaspoon vanilla extract	¼ teaspoon salt
1 cup all-purpose flour	

1. Preheat oven to 350°F. Grease a 9-inch square pan. In a medium bowl, beat oil, honey, and sugar with an electric mixer on medium speed until well blended. Beat in eggs and vanilla until light and fluffy.

2. In another bowl, mix all-purpose flour, whole wheat flour, baking powder, baking soda, cinnamon, and salt. Beat in on low speed until a soft dough forms, scraping down side of bowl frequently with a rubber spatula. Turn into prepared pan and level surface.

3. Bake 20 to 22 minutes, or until top is golden brown and a toothpick inserted in center comes out clean. Remove pan to a rack and cut into 16 squares. Store in a tightly covered container.

194 CINNAMON BLONDIES
Prep: 10 minutes   Bake: 20 to 25 minutes   Makes: 16

¾ cup flour	1 stick (4 ounces) butter,
½ teaspoon baking powder	softened
1 tablespoon cinnamon	2 eggs
¼ teaspoon salt	1 teaspoon vanilla extract
¾ cup sugar	½ cup chopped walnuts

1. Preheat oven to 350°F. Grease a 9-inch square pan. In a medium bowl, stir together flour, baking powder, cinnamon, and salt.

2. In a large bowl, beat sugar and butter with an electric mixer on medium speed until fluffy. Add eggs and vanilla and beat until smooth. Add flour mixture and beat on low speed until a soft dough forms, scraping down side of bowl frequently with a rubber spatula. Fold in walnuts. Turn dough into prepared pan, leveling surface.

3. Bake 20 to 25 minutes, or until top is golden brown and a toothpick inserted in center comes out clean. Remove pan to a rack and cut into 16 squares. Store in a tightly covered container.

195 CORNMEAL-CHIP BLONDIES
Prep: 10 minutes   Bake: 18 to 20 minutes   Makes: 32

Cornmeal adds a sweet nutty crunch to these crisp blondies.

¾ cup flour	1 stick (4 ounces) butter,
⅔ cup yellow cornmeal	softened
½ teaspoon baking powder	½ cup sugar
¼ teaspoon salt	1 tablespoon vanilla extract
	½ cup mini chocolate chips

1. Preheat oven to 350°F. Grease two 8-inch square pans. In a medium bowl, stir together flour, cornmeal, baking powder, and salt.

2. In a large bowl, beat butter, sugar, and vanilla with an electric mixer on medium speed until smooth. Add flour mixture and beat on low speed until a stiff, crumbly dough forms, scraping down side of bowl frequently with a rubber spatula. Fold in chocolate chips. Divide dough between prepared pans, patting to level surface.

3. Bake 18 to 20 minutes, or until tops are golden brown and a toothpick inserted in center of each comes out clean. Remove pans to a rack, cut each into 16 squares, and let cool completely. Store in an airtight container or wrap well and refrigerate.

Chapter 8

Eve's Temptation

There is more than one way to enjoy the valuable nutrients, high fiber, and delicious flavor of fruit. Of course, there are lots of ways, but we think fruit bars are one of the best. Thrifty cooks have always added fruit in season to their cakes and cookies to extend the more expensive ingredients, such as sugar and shortening. As an added bonus, they found that fruit-filled baked products stayed moist longer and added variety to their menus.

Whether they use fresh, dried, or preserved fruit, fruit bars are particularly easy to make. They can be spread or patted into a pan, then baked, cut, and stored in the same pan. There is no rolling out, cutting, removing to cooling racks, or packing into storage containers. The only care necessary in their preparation is to make sure the baking pan size is correct and that the batter or dough is spread evenly into the pan, so it will all be finished baking at the same time. Another important tip is to check your bars at the minimum baking time. If you are using dark baking pans, the bars will bake faster.

Because they are moist, fruit bars are good travelers. If you are bringing them to an event, they can be carried right in their baking pan.

If you are looking for variety in your cookie jar and a way to add at least some extra potassium and fiber, fruit bars are a good choice. They come in a wide spectrum of enticing colors and flavors. Don't stop with just Eve's apple; tempt your family and friends with apricot, cherry, date, banana, and raisin as well.

196   APPLE BUTTER BARS
Prep: 10 minutes   Bake: 20 to 25 minutes   Makes: 20

It's the apple butter that gives these cakelike bars their delectable flavor.

4 tablespoons butter, softened	½ teaspoon baking soda
½ cup firmly packed dark brown sugar	¼ teaspoon salt
	¾ cup apple butter
1 egg	½ cup chopped walnuts
½ teaspoon vanilla extract	½ cup golden raisins
1 cup flour	¼ cup powdered sugar

1. Preheat oven to 350°F. Grease a 9-inch square pan. In a large bowl, beat butter and brown sugar with an electric mixer on medium speed until light and fluffy. Beat in egg and vanilla.

2. Add flour mixed with baking soda and salt and beat on low speed until blended. With a large spoon, stir in apple butter, walnuts, and raisins. Turn batter into prepared pan, leveling surface.

3. Bake 20 to 25 minutes, until a toothpick inserted in center comes out with a few moist crumbs clinging to it. Remove to a rack. Let cool completely in pan. Sprinkle with powdered sugar and cut into 20 bars before serving.

---

197   APPLESAUCE BARS
Prep: 10 minutes   Bake: 25 to 30 minutes   Makes: 20

1⅓ cups flour	⅔ cup firmly packed brown sugar
1 teaspoon baking powder	
¼ teaspoon baking soda	1 egg
1 teaspoon cinnamon	1 cup unsweetened applesauce
½ teaspoon ground ginger	
¼ teaspoon grated nutmeg	½ cup chopped walnuts
¼ teaspoon salt	½ cup raisins
4 tablespoons butter, softened	

1. Preheat oven to 350°F. Grease a 9-inch square pan. In a medium bowl, stir together flour, baking powder, baking soda, cinnamon, ginger, nutmeg, and salt.

2. In a large bowl, beat butter, brown sugar, and egg with an electric mixer on medium speed until smooth. Add applesauce and flour mixture and beat on low speed just until batter is smooth, scraping down side of bowl frequently with a rubber spatula. Fold in nuts and raisins. Turn batter into prepared pan, leveling surface.

3. Bake 25 to 30 minutes, or until top is golden brown and a toothpick inserted in center comes out clean. Remove pan to a rack, cut into 20 bars, and let cool completely. Store in an airtight container in refrigerator.

198 ALMOND CHERRY BARS
Prep: 15 minutes   Bake: 25 to 30 minutes   Makes: 20

4 tablespoons butter, softened
1 cup firmly packed dark
   brown sugar
1 egg
1 teaspoon vanilla extract
¾ cup flour
½ teaspoon baking powder

¼ teaspoon salt
⅓ cup cherry preserves
½ cup dried cherries
½ cup chopped almonds
½ cup powdered sugar
1 to 2 tablespoons kirsch or
   brandy

1. Preheat oven to 350°F. Grease an 8-inch square pan. In a medium bowl, beat butter and brown sugar with an electric mixer on medium speed until light and fluffy. Beat in egg and vanilla until blended. Add flour mixed with baking powder and salt and beat until blended.

2. In a small bowl, stir together cherry preserves, dried cherries, and chopped almonds until blended. Mix into dough.

3. Spread into prepared pan. Bake 25 to 30 minutes, or until golden. Remove to a rack and let cool completely.

4. Mix powdered sugar with enough kirsch to make a thick glaze; drizzle over top. Cut into 20 bars.

199 APPLE MINCEMEAT BARS
Prep: 15 minutes   Bake: 25 to 30 minutes   Makes: 27

6 tablespoons butter, softened
½ cup firmly packed dark
   brown sugar
½ cup mincemeat
¾ cup flour
½ cup rolled oats

½ teaspoon baking soda
¼ teaspoon salt
1 cup finely chopped, peeled
   tart apple, such as Granny
   Smith
⅓ cup chopped walnuts

1. Preheat oven to 350°F. Grease an 8-inch square pan. In a medium bowl, beat butter and brown sugar with an electric mixer on medium speed until creamy. On low speed, beat in mincemeat until well blended.

2. Add flour mixed with oatmeal, baking soda, and salt and beat until well blended. Stir in chopped apple and walnuts.

3. Press dough into prepared pan, being careful to level surface. Bake 25 to 30 minutes, until a toothpick inserted in center comes out with a few moist crumbs clinging to it. Remove pan to a rack and let cool completely before cutting into 27 bars.

200   APPLE WALNUT BARS
Prep: 12 minutes   Bake: 30 to 35 minutes   Makes: 27

1 large Granny Smith apple
1 cup rolled oats
¾ cup graham cracker crumbs
4 tablespoons butter, softened
3 tablespoons sugar

1 cup chopped walnuts
½ cup flaked coconut
1 (14-ounce) can sweetened
     condensed milk

1. Preheat oven to 350°F. Peel, core, and finely chop apple. There should be about 1½ cups.

2. In a medium bowl, stir together oatmeal, graham cracker crumbs, butter, and sugar until blended. Press firmly into bottom of a greased 9-inch square pan.

3. Top with chopped apples, walnuts, and coconut. Pour condensed milk over top.

4. Bake 30 to 35 minutes, until lightly browned. Remove pan to a rack and let cool completely before cutting into 27 bars.

201   FIRST DATE BARS
Prep: 15 minutes   Bake: 20 to 25 minutes   Makes: 20

Orange, dates, nuts, and chocolate offer just about everything you might wish for in a bar cookie.

1 cup flour
1 teaspoon baking powder
1 teaspoon grated orange zest
¼ teaspoon salt
1 cup chopped dates
4 tablespoons butter, softened
1 cup firmly packed dark
     brown sugar

2 eggs
2 tablespoons orange juice
1 teaspoon vanilla extract
½ cup chopped nuts
½ cup semisweet chocolate
     chips

1. Preheat oven to 350°F. Grease a 9-inch square pan. In a small bowl, stir together flour, baking powder, orange zest, and salt. Remove 1 tablespoon of flour mixture and toss with dates.

2. In a large bowl, beat butter and brown sugar with an electric mixer on medium speed until fluffy. Beat in eggs, orange juice, and vanilla until smooth.

3. Add flour mixture and beat on low speed until dough is smooth, scraping down side of bowl frequently with a rubber spatula. Stir in dates, nuts, and chocolate chips. Turn into prepared pan, being careful to level surface.

4. Bake 20 to 25 minutes, until a toothpick inserted in center comes out with a few moist crumbs clinging to it. Remove pan to rack. Let cool completely in pan before cutting into 20 bars.

202   CRANBERRY BARS
Prep: 10 minutes   Bake: 27 to 32 minutes   Makes: 24

These bars will delight cranberry lovers. They're filled not only with tart dried cranberries, but with walnuts and coconut as well.

   4   tablespoons butter, softened
   ¼   cup firmly packed dark
        brown sugar
   ½   cup plus 2 tablespoons flour
   1   egg
   ½   cup granulated sugar
   ¾   cup dried cranberries (about
        3 ounces)

   ½   cup chopped walnuts
   ½   cup flaked coconut
   1   tablespoon Grand Marnier
        or orange juice
   1   teaspoon grated orange zest
   ½   teaspoon vanilla extract
   ¼   teaspoon salt

1. Preheat oven to 350°F. In a medium bowl, stir together butter, brown sugar, and ½ cup flour until blended. Press firmly into bottom of an ungreased 8-inch square pan. Bake 7 minutes.

2. Meanwhile, combine remaining 2 tablespoons flour with egg, granulated sugar, dried cranberries, walnuts, coconut, Grand Marnier, orange zest, vanilla, and salt. Stir well to mix. Carefully spread over warm crust and return to oven.

3. Bake 20 to 25 minutes, until edges are lightly browned. Remove pan to a rack and let cool completely before cutting into 24 bars.

203   APRICOT BARS
Prep: 15 minutes   Bake: 35 to 40 minutes   Makes: 18

Our friend Chris Koury shared her delicious apricot bars with us.

   1½   sticks (6 ounces) butter,
         softened
   ½   cup granulated sugar
   ⅓   cup firmly packed light
         brown sugar

   2   cups flour
   ¼   teaspoon baking soda
   ¼   teaspoon salt
   ¾   cup apricot preserves
   1   tablespoon lemon juice

1. Preheat oven to 350°F. Grease a 9-inch square pan. In a medium bowl, beat butter until creamy with an electric mixer on medium speed. Beat in granulated sugar and brown sugar. Stir in flour mixed with baking soda and salt until crumbly.

2. Measure out and reserve 1 cup crumb mixture. Press remainder over bottom of prepared pan.

3. In a small bowl, stir together apricot preserves and lemon juice. Spread into pan, leaving a ¼-inch border all around edges. Sprinkle remaining crumbs evenly on top.

4. Bake 35 to 40 minutes, until lightly browned. Remove pan to a wire rack and let cool completely before cutting into 18 bars.

204   DREAMY DATE-NUT BARS
Prep: 10 minutes   Bake: 25 to 32 minutes   Makes: 24

4 tablespoons butter, softened
⅓ cup plus 1 tablespoon flour
1¼ cups firmly packed dark
    brown sugar
1 egg
1 teaspoon vanilla extract

½ teaspoon baking powder
¼ teaspoon salt
1 cup chopped dates
1 cup chopped walnuts
1 cup flaked coconut

1. Preheat oven to 350°F. In a large bowl, beat butter, ⅓ cup flour, and ¼ cup brown sugar with an electric mixer on medium speed until blended. Press into an ungreased 8-inch square pan. Bake 10 to 12 minutes, until edges brown.

2. Meanwhile, in a medium bowl, beat egg with an electric mixer on medium speed until fluffy. Add remaining 1 cup brown sugar and beat until light and fluffy. Blend in vanilla, remaining 1 tablespoon flour, baking powder, and salt. Stir in dates, walnuts, and coconut.

3. Spread date-nut topping over warm crust and return to oven. Bake 15 to 20 minutes, or until topping is set and lightly browned. Remove pan to a rack and let cool completely before cutting into 24 bars.

205   FRUIT 'N' HONEY BARS
Prep: 10 minutes   Bake: 40 to 45 minutes   Makes: 20

As with all baked goods made with honey, these mellow and become more flavorful the day after they're baked.

1 stick (4 ounces) butter,
    softened
⅓ cup honey
2 eggs
¾ cup flour
½ teaspoon baking powder
½ teaspoon salt

½ cup raisins
½ cup flaked coconut
½ cup chopped walnuts
¼ cup currants
¼ cup golden raisins
2 tablespoons powdered
    sugar

1. Preheat oven to 300°F. Grease an 8-inch square pan. In a medium bowl, beat butter and honey with electric mixer on medium speed until creamy. Beat in eggs until well blended.

2. Add flour mixed with baking powder and salt and beat until blended. Stir in raisins, coconut, walnuts, currants, and golden raisins. Turn into prepared pan, leveling surface.

3. Bake 40 to 45 minutes, until a cake tester inserted in center comes out clean. Remove to a rack and let cool completely before cutting into 20 bars. Sprinkle powdered sugar on top before serving.

206 CHUNKY CHERRY CHEWS
Prep: 10 minutes   Bake: 25 to 30 minutes   Makes: 42

1 stick (4 ounces) butter, softened	½ teaspoon baking powder
½ cup firmly packed dark brown sugar	¼ teaspoon salt
½ cup granulated sugar	1½ cups walnuts
1 egg	1 cup golden raisins
½ teaspoon vanilla extract	6 ounces dried cherries, sweet or sour
1½ cups rolled oats	1 (14-ounce) can sweetened condensed milk
1¼ cups flour	

1. Preheat oven to 350°F. Grease a 9 × 13-inch baking pan. In a large bowl, beat butter with brown sugar and granulated sugar with an electric mixer on medium speed until light and fluffy. Beat in egg and vanilla until well blended.

2. Add oatmeal mixed with flour, baking powder, and salt and stir well. Reserve one cup of dough; press remainder into bottom of prepared baking pan.

3. Sprinkle walnuts, golden raisins, and dried cherries evenly over dough. Pour condensed milk on top. Crumble reserved dough over condensed milk.

4. Bake 25 to 30 minutes, until lightly browned. Remove pan to a rack and let cool completely before cutting into 42 bars.

207 DATE DOTS
Prep: 7 minutes   Bake: 20 to 22 minutes   Makes: 25

These little date squares stay soft and chewy for up to a week at room temperature, making them an excellent choice for mailing.

1 cup powdered sugar	1 tablespoon butter, softened
1 cup pitted dates	¼ cup flour
1 cup walnuts	½ teaspoon cinnamon
2 eggs	¼ teaspoon salt

1. Preheat oven to 350°F. Set aside 1 tablespoon powdered sugar. In a food processor, combine remaining powdered sugar with dates, walnuts, eggs, butter, flour, cinnamon, and salt. Process until dates and nuts are finely chopped.

2. Turn date mixture into a greased 9-inch square pan, leveling surface. Bake 20 to 22 minutes, or until center is firm.

3. While still warm, cut into 25 squares and sift reserved powdered sugar over top. Place on a wire rack and let cool completely. Store in an airtight container.

208 LEBKUCHEN BARS
Prep: 10 minutes   Bake: 25 to 30 minutes   Makes: 24

This easy-to-make version of the European holiday cookie is good for lunch boxes and snacks all year round.

1½ cups firmly packed brown sugar	½ teaspoon baking soda
2 eggs	¼ teaspoon ground cloves
2 teaspoons vanilla extract	1 cup finely chopped walnuts
1¾ cups flour	¼ cup citron, finely chopped
1 teaspoon cinnamon	¼ cup raisins, chopped
½ teaspoon baking powder	½ cup powdered sugar
	1 tablespoon brandy

1. Preheat oven to 350°F. Grease a 9 × 13-inch baking pan. In a medium bowl, beat brown sugar, eggs, and vanilla with an electric mixer on high speed until fluffy.

2. Add flour mixed with cinnamon, baking powder, baking soda, and cloves; beat on low speed until a soft dough forms, scraping down side of bowl frequently with a rubber spatula. Fold walnuts, citron, and raisins into dough. Turn dough into prepared pan, leveling surface.

3. Bake 25 to 30 minutes, or until top is golden brown and a toothpick inserted in center comes out clean. Remove pan to a rack and cut into 24 bars.

4. Combine powdered sugar and brandy; spread over bars. Set aside to cool completely. Store in an airtight container.

209 APRICOT ALMOND BARS
Prep: 10 minutes   Bake: 20 to 25 minutes   Makes: 25

For a change once in a while, try this recipe with peach or mango preserves in place of the apricot.

2 cups flour	1 teaspoon vanilla extract
2 teaspoons baking powder	½ teaspoon almond extract
¼ teaspoon salt	⅔ cup apricot preserves
½ cup sugar	¼ cup finely chopped dried apricots
4 tablespoons butter, melted	¼ cup sliced almonds
2 eggs	

1. Preheat oven to 350°F. Grease a 9 × 13-inch baking pan. In a small bowl, stir together flour, baking powder, and salt.

2. In a large bowl, beat sugar and butter with an electric mixer on medium speed until fluffy. Beat in eggs, one at a time, until very fluffy. Beat in vanilla and almond extract.

3. Add flour mixture to sugar mixture; beat on low speed until dough is smooth, scraping down side of bowl frequently with a rubber spatula. Spread two thirds of dough into bottom of prepared pan, leveling surface. Combine apricot preserves and dried apricots; spread evenly over dough. With floured fingers, pull remaining dough into small pieces and drop over preserves, allowing some spots to remain uncovered. Sprinkle almonds on top.

4. Bake 20 to 25 minutes, or until top is golden brown and a toothpick inserted in center comes out with a few moist crumbs clinging to it. Remove pan to a rack, cut into 25 bars, and let cool completely. Store in an airtight container or wrap well and refrigerate.

---

210   LINZER BARS
Prep: 25 minutes   Bake: 20 to 25 minutes   Makes: 20

Serve this cookie version of the famous Viennese linzertorte with a cup of whipped cream–topped Viennese coffee. For a less sweet version, use raspberry fruit spread in place of the preserves.

½ cup firmly packed light
    brown sugar
1 stick (4 ounces) butter,
    softened
1 egg
1 teaspoon vanilla extract
¾ cup all-purpose flour
½ cup whole wheat flour

½ cup finely chopped
    hazelnuts or pecans
½ teaspoon cinnamon
¼ teaspoon baking powder
¼ teaspoon salt
¾ cup seedless red raspberry
    preserves
Powdered sugar

1. Preheat oven to 350°F. Grease a 9 × 13-inch baking pan.

2. In a large bowl, beat brown sugar and butter with an electric mixer on medium speed until fluffy. Beat in egg and vanilla until smooth. In a small bowl, combine all-purpose flour, whole wheat flour, nuts, cinnamon, baking powder, and salt. Add to sugar-butter mixture and beat on low speed until a soft dough forms, scraping down side of bowl frequently with a rubber spatula.

3. Remove ⅔ cup of dough and place in a pastry bag fitted with ¼-inch open tip or a parchment cone with the tip cut off to make a ¼-inch opening. Pat remaining dough into bottom of prepared baking pan. Gently spread raspberry preserves over dough. With pastry bag or plastic bag, pipe 5 strips of reserved dough diagonally crosswise on top of preserves. Pipe 5 more strips diagonally crosswise in other direction.

4. Bake 20 to 25 minutes, or until top crust is golden brown. Remove pan to a rack, cut into 20 bars, and let cool completely. Store in an airtight container or wrap well and refrigerate. Dust bars with powdered sugar just before serving.

211 OATMEAL BANANA BARS
Prep: 10 minutes   Bake: 25 to 30 minutes   Makes: 12

This is a soft, moist bar. For best flavor, use very ripe bananas that are well spotted with brown.

6 tablespoons butter, softened	¼ teaspoon salt
½ cup firmly packed dark brown sugar	2 cups quick-cooking rolled oats
1 cup mashed ripe bananas (about 2 medium)	¼ cup golden raisins
	¼ cup dark raisins
1 egg	½ cup toasted slivered almonds

1. Preheat oven to 350°F. Grease a 9-inch square pan. In a medium bowl, beat butter and brown sugar with an electric mixer on medium speed until creamy. Add mashed bananas, egg, and salt and beat until well blended.

2. Stir in oatmeal, golden and dark raisins, and almonds. Spread batter evenly in prepared pan.

3. Bake 25 to 30 minutes, or until a cake tester inserted in center comes out clean. Let cool on rack completely before cutting into 12 bars.

---

212 OATMEAL DATE SQUARES
Prep: 10 minutes   Bake: 25 to 30 minutes   Makes: 16

Tuck a few of these high-energy cookies in your pocket when you go for a hike or bike ride.

½ cup flour	⅓ cup firmly packed brown sugar
1 teaspoon cinnamon	
½ teaspoon baking powder	1 egg
⅛ teaspoon salt	1 teaspoon vanilla extract
1 stick (4 ounces) butter, softened	1 cup rolled oats
	½ cup chopped dates

1. Preheat oven to 350°F. Grease an 8-inch square pan. In a small bowl, stir together flour, cinnamon, baking powder, and salt.

2. In a large bowl, beat butter and brown sugar with an electric mixer on medium speed until fluffy. Beat in egg and vanilla until smooth.

3. Add flour mixture. Beat on low speed until a soft dough forms, scraping down side of bowl frequently with a rubber spatula. Fold oats and dates into dough. Turn dough into prepared pan, leveling surface.

4. Bake 25 to 30 minutes, or until top is golden brown and a toothpick inserted in center comes out clean. Remove pan to a rack, cut into 16 squares, and let cool completely. Store in an airtight container or wrap well and refrigerate.

213 RAISIN SQUARES

Prep: 15 minutes   Chill: 10 minutes   Bake: 12 to 15 minutes
Makes: 16

1   stick (4 ounces) butter,
    softened
¼   cup sugar
1   egg
1   tablespoon lemon juice
1   teaspoon grated lemon zest
1½ cups flour
¼   teaspoon baking powder

¼   teaspoon salt
1   cup muscat raisins or regular
    raisins
1   tablespoon brown sugar
¼   teaspoon cinnamon
¼   teaspoon ground ginger
⅛   teaspoon grated nutmeg

1. Preheat oven to 350°F. In a medium bowl, beat butter and sugar with an electric mixer on medium speed until well blended. Beat in egg, lemon juice, and lemon zest until light and fluffy.

2. Add flour mixed with baking powder and salt and beat on low speed until a stiff dough forms, scraping down side of bowl frequently with a rubber spatula. Divide dough in half.

3. Between pieces of wax paper, roll out half of dough about ⅛ inch thick to make a 10-inch square. Place on baking sheet, still between sheets of wax paper, and place in freezer 10 minutes. Place remaining half of dough on a lightly greased cookie sheet, cover with a sheet of wax paper, and roll to make another 10-inch square. Remove wax paper.

4. Toss raisins with a mixture of brown sugar, cinnamon, ginger, and nutmeg. Sprinkle evenly over dough on cookie sheet. Remove dough square from freezer. Peel off one sheet of wax paper. Using remaining wax paper for support, invert over dough and raisins on cookie sheet so that edges match edges of other dough square. With wax paper still on top, roll over dough with a rolling pin to seal; peel off and discard wax paper. With a moistened long sharp knife, cut into 16 (2½-inch) squares but do not separate. With tines of a fork, pierce center of each square.

5. Bake squares 12 to 15 minutes, or until golden brown. Remove to a rack and let cool completely. Break into 16 squares where cut and store in a tightly covered container.

214 RAISIN-SPICE BARS

Prep: 10 minutes   Bake: 20 to 25 minutes   Makes: 16

½ cup flour
½ teaspoon baking powder
¼ teaspoon baking soda
1½ teaspoons grated nutmeg
1 teaspoon cinnamon
¼ teaspoon ground allspice
⅛ teaspoon salt
   Pinch of ground cloves
4 tablespoons butter,
   softened

¼ cup firmly packed brown
   sugar
½ cup light corn syrup
1 egg
1 teaspoon vanilla extract
½ cup rolled oats
1 cup raisins
½ cup coarsely chopped nuts

1. Preheat oven to 350°F. Grease an 8-inch square pan. In a small bowl, stir together flour, baking powder, baking soda, nutmeg, cinnamon, allspice, salt, and cloves until well mixed.

2. In a large bowl, beat butter and brown sugar with an electric mixer on medium speed until fluffy. Beat in corn syrup, then egg and vanilla until smooth.

3. Add flour mixture and beat on low speed until dough is smooth, scraping down side of bowl frequently with a rubber spatula. Stir in oatmeal, raisins, and nuts. Turn into prepared pan, leveling surface.

4. Bake 20 to 25 minutes, until a toothpick inserted in center comes out with a few moist crumbs clinging to it. Remove pan to a rack. Let cool completely in pan before cutting into 16 bars.

Chapter 9

Other Squares and Bars

This chapter includes all those squares and bars that aren't brownies, blondies, or filled with fruit. Most are prepared and baked in the same manner as the ones in the previous three chapters, and they share the same concerns about using the correct pan sizes, baking times, and tests to make sure they are baked to perfection.

Except for those recipes in which we recommend refrigeration because they contain perishable products, bars are a very good choice for mailing to family and friends away from home. Along with soft drop cookies, they travel well because they are moist and more resilient to the jarring encountered in the mail.

Wrap bars or cookies individually or no more than four to a packet, and layer them in a box that has been completely lined with plastic wrap or aluminum foil. For a natural and edible packing material, fill all empty spaces in the box with popped corn or puffed wheat. And when baking treats to mail away, be sure to put an extra batch in the oven for the family.

215 CARAMEL OATMEAL SQUARES
Prep: 15 minutes   Bake: 18 to 22 minutes   Makes: 25

1 stick (4 ounces) butter,
   softened
1 cup sugar
1 egg
½ teaspoon vanilla extract
1½ cups rolled oats
1¼ cups flour
½ teaspoon baking powder

¼ teaspoon baking soda
½ teaspoon salt
½ teaspoon cinnamon
½ cup semisweet chocolate
   chips
12 soft caramel squares (about
   3½ ounces)

1. Preheat oven to 375°F. In a medium bowl, beat butter and sugar with an electric mixer on medium speed until fluffy. Beat in egg until well blended, then beat in vanilla. Mix oatmeal and flour with baking powder, baking soda, salt, and cinnamon. Stir in and beat until well blended. Press half of dough into an ungreased 8-inch square pan. Sprinkle chocolate chips over top.

2. In a microwave-safe bowl, combine caramels and 2 teaspoons water. Microwave at 50 percent power 2 to 3 minutes, stirring occasionally, until caramels melt. Drizzle over chocolate chips. Crumble remaining dough over top.

3. Bake 18 to 22 minutes, until top is lightly browned. Remove to a rack and let cool completely before cutting into 25 squares.

---

216 ALMOND BARS
Prep: 15 minutes   Bake: 20 to 25 minutes   Makes: 20

1 stick (4 ounces) butter,
   softened
½ teaspoon vanilla extract
½ teaspoon almond extract
¼ teaspoon salt

½ cup sugar
1 cup flour
½ cup semisweet chocolate
   chips
½ cup chopped almonds

1. Preheat oven to 350°F. In a large bowl, beat butter, vanilla, almond extract, and salt with an electric mixer on medium speed until creamy. Gradually beat in sugar and continue beating until light and fluffy.

2. Fold in flour and chocolate chips. With a rubber scraper, turn batter into an ungreased 9-inch square pan, leveling surface. Sprinkle almonds over batter and gently press in.

3. Bake 20 to 25 minutes, or until golden. Remove pan to rack, cut into 20 bars, and let cool completely in pan.

217 UNBELIEVABLY ALMONDY ALMOND BARS

Prep: 10 minutes   Bake: 25 to 30 minutes   Makes: 24

1 stick (4 ounces) butter, softened	1 tablespoon Amaretto, or other almond-flavored liqueur
3½ ounces almond paste (about ⅓ cup)	1 teaspoon vanilla extract
1 cup firmly packed dark brown sugar	¼ teaspoon salt
1 egg	1¼ cups flour
	¾ cup chopped almonds

1. Preheat oven to 350°F. Grease a 9-inch square pan. In a medium bowl, beat butter, almond paste, and brown sugar with electric mixer on medium speed until creamy. Beat in egg, Amaretto, vanilla, and salt.

2. Stir in flour and ½ cup chopped almonds. Turn into prepared pan, leveling surface. Sprinkle remaining ¼ cup nuts over top.

3. Bake 25 to 30 minutes, or until a toothpick inserted in center comes out with a few moist crumbs clinging to it. Remove to a rack and let cool completely before cutting into 24 bars.

218 CHEESECAKE SQUARES

Prep: 15 minutes   Bake: 20 to 22 minutes   Makes: 16

For a quick-to-make company dessert, cut these into six rectangles and top with fresh berries.

½ cup powdered sugar	1 (8-ounce) package cream cheese, softened
4 tablespoons butter, softened	¼ cup granulated sugar
¾ cup flour	1 egg
¼ cup finely ground natural almonds	½ teaspoon almond extract
¼ teaspoon salt	

1. Preheat oven to 350°F. Grease a 9-inch square pan.

2. In a medium bowl, beat together powdered sugar and butter with a hand-held electric mixer on medium speed until well blended. Add flour, almonds, and salt. Beat on low speed until dough is smooth, scraping down side of bowl frequently with a rubber spatula. Turn dough into prepared pan. With floured fingers, pat gently against bottom of pan to make an even crust. Bake 10 minutes; crust will be partially baked.

3. Meanwhile, in same bowl, with electric mixer on medium speed, beat together cream cheese, granulated sugar, egg, and almond extract until smooth. Spread mixture evenly over partially baked crust.

4. Return to oven and bake 10 to 12 minutes longer, until top is set and lightly browned. Remove pan to a rack, cut into 16 squares, and let cool completely. Wrap well and refrigerate.

219 CHOCOLATE CARAMEL CRUNCH BARS
Prep: 20 minutes   Cook: 5 to 6 minutes   Makes: 48

2 sticks (8 ounces) butter, melted
1 cup sugar
½ cup unsweetened cocoa powder
1 tablespoon vanilla extract
4 cups chocolate wafer cookie crumbs (about 36 cookies)
½ cup finely chopped pecans

2 (14-ounce) cans sweetened condensed milk (*not* evaporated milk)
4 tablespoons butter
¼ cup plus 2 tablespoons light corn syrup
12 ounces semisweet chocolate chips (2 cups)

1. Grease a 10 × 15-inch jelly-roll pan. In a medium bowl, stir together melted butter, sugar, cocoa powder, 2 teaspoons vanilla, cookie crumbs, and nuts. Press evenly into bottom of prepared pan.

2. In a small saucepan, heat condensed milk, butter, and corn syrup over medium-high heat until mixture comes to a boil. Boil 3 minutes, stirring constantly. Remove from heat, stir in remaining 1 teaspoon vanilla, and pour evenly over crumb layer. Let cool completely.

3. Melt chocolate chips in a microwave or in a double boiler over simmering water, stirring until melted and smooth, 2 to 3 minutes. Remove from heat and let cool slightly. Spread melted chocolate over top. Let cool until chocolate is set. Cut into 48 bars.

220 CHOCOLATE HAZELNUT BARS
Prep: 15 minutes   Bake: 10 minutes   Makes: 16

1 stick (4 ounces) butter, softened
¾ cup firmly packed dark brown sugar
1½ cups flour
⅛ teaspoon salt

½ cup finely ground toasted hazelnuts
6 ounces semisweet chocolate chips (1 cup)
¼ cup light corn syrup
2 tablespoons orange juice

1. Preheat oven to 350°F. In a medium bowl, beat butter and brown sugar with an electric mixer on medium speed until blended. Beat in flour and salt until thoroughly combined. Press evenly into bottom of an 8-inch square baking pan. Bake 10 minutes, or until lightly browned. Remove to a rack. Sprinkle ¼ cup ground hazelnuts over crust.

2. Meanwhile, in a small saucepan, combine chocolate chips, corn syrup, and orange juice. Cook over medium heat, stirring, until chocolate melts, about 2 minutes. Bring to a boil and cook 1 minute. Remove from heat and pour over crust.

3. Sprinkle remaining ¼ cup hazelnuts over top. Let cool completely before cutting into 16 bars.

221 PEANUT BUTTER BARS
Prep: 10 minutes   Bake: 20 to 25 minutes   Makes: 20

¾ cup flour
1 teaspoon baking powder
⅛ teaspoon salt
½ cup chunky peanut butter
4 tablespoons butter, softened
½ cup firmly packed dark
   brown sugar

¼ cup granulated sugar
2 eggs
1 teaspoon vanilla extract
⅔ cup semisweet chocolate
   chips

1. Preheat oven to 350°F. Grease a 9-inch square pan. In a small bowl, stir together flour, baking powder, and salt.

2. In a large bowl, beat peanut butter and butter with an electric mixer on medium speed until creamy. Add brown sugar and granulated sugar and beat until well blended. Beat in eggs and vanilla until well blended.

3. Add flour mixture and beat on low speed until dough is smooth, scraping down side of bowl frequently with a rubber spatula. Fold in chocolate chips. Turn dough into prepared pan, leveling surface.

4. Bake 20 to 25 minutes, until a toothpick inserted in center comes out with a few moist crumbs clinging to it. Remove pan to a rack. Let cool completely in pan before cutting into 20 bars.

222 CRUNCHY JAM SQUARES
Prep: 15 minutes   Bake: 25 to 30 minutes   Makes: 36

This is a snap to make in your food processor.

1¼ cups rolled oats
¾ cup all-purpose flour
½ cup whole wheat flour
1 cup firmly packed dark
   brown sugar
¼ cup flaked coconut
1 stick (4 ounces) plus
   2 tablespoons butter,
   chilled and cut into pieces

¼ teaspoon salt
½ cup chopped almonds
⅔ cup strawberry jam
2 tablespoons framboise,
   kirsch, or raspberry
   brandy

1. Preheat oven to 375°F. In a food processor, combine oatmeal, all-purpose flour, whole wheat flour, brown sugar, coconut, butter, and salt. Pulse until crumbly. Press two thirds of dough in bottom of a greased 9-inch square pan. Mix almonds into remaining dough.

2. In a small bowl, stir together jam and liqueur. Spread over dough, then top with remaining dough. Press gently.

3. Bake 25 to 30 minutes, until golden brown. Remove to a wire rack and let cool completely before cutting into 36 squares.

223   CREAMY DREAMY CHOCOLATE BARS
Prep: 10 minutes   Bake: 28 to 30 minutes   Makes: 40

This moist, chewy brownie stuffed with chocolate is sure to become a family favorite.

2¼ cups flour
1 cup sugar
¾ cup rolled oats
⅓ cup unsweetened cocoa powder
½ teaspoon baking soda
½ teaspoon salt
2 sticks (8 ounces) butter, melted

1 egg, slightly beaten
2 teaspoons vanilla extract
1 (14-ounce) can sweetened condensed milk (*not* evaporated milk)
6 ounces semisweet chocolate chips (1 cup)

1. Preheat oven to 375°F. Grease a 9 × 13-inch baking pan. In a medium bowl, stir together flour, sugar, oatmeal, cocoa powder, baking soda, and salt until blended. Mix in melted butter, egg, and vanilla until mixture resembles coarse crumbs. Set aside 1½ cups. Press remaining mixture into bottom of prepared pan.

2. Bake 10 minutes. Remove from oven and leave oven on. Pour condensed milk over crust to within ½ inch of edge. Sprinkle chocolate chips and reserved crumbs evenly over milk, pressing in lightly. Bake an additional 18 to 20 minutes, or until set. Remove to a rack and let cool thoroughly before cutting into 40 bars.

---

224   COCONUT MARSHMALLOW BARS
Prep: 15 minutes   Bake: 18 to 20 minutes   Makes: 25

Melted marshmallows make a quick topping for these bars.

⅓ cup sugar
6 tablespoons butter, melted
1 egg
2 teaspoons vanilla extract
¾ cup flour

¾ teaspoon baking powder
⅛ teaspoon salt
1 cup flaked coconut
1 (10-ounce) package marshmallows

1. Preheat oven to 350°F. Grease a 9 × 13-inch baking pan.

2. In a large bowl, beat sugar and 4 tablespoons butter with an electric mixer on medium speed until fluffy. Beat in egg and 1 teaspoon vanilla until very fluffy.

3. Add flour mixed with baking powder and salt to sugar mixture. Beat on low speed until dough is smooth, scraping down side of bowl frequently with a rubber spatula. Spread dough over bottom of prepared pan, leveling surface with a rubber scraper.

4. Bake 18 to 20 minutes, or until top is golden brown and a toothpick inserted in center comes out clean. Remove pan to a rack.

5. Meanwhile, place coconut on a baking sheet and toast in oven 6 to 8 minutes, stirring occasionally, until golden brown.

6. In a medium saucepan, warm marshmallows and remaining 2 tablespoons butter over very low heat, stirring occasionally, until melted. Remove from heat and stir in remaining 1 teaspoon vanilla. Pour over cookie crust; sprinkle with toasted coconut and set aside 2 to 3 hours to cool completely.

7. To serve, cut into 25 bars with a moist knife. Store between layers of wax paper in a tightly covered container. If bars are cut before completely cool, marshmallow will spread together and will need to be recut once cool in order to separate completely.

---

225   LEMON BITES
Prep: 15 minutes   Bake: 45 to 50 minutes   Makes: 30

1 stick (4 ounces) butter, softened
¼ cup firmly packed dark brown sugar
1 cup plus 2 tablespoons flour
1 teaspoon grated lemon zest
¼ teaspoon lemon extract (optional)

2 eggs
1¼ cups plus 2 tablespoons powdered sugar
½ teaspoon baking powder
Juice of 1 lemon (about 3 tablespoons)

1. Preheat oven to 350°F. In a large bowl, beat butter and brown sugar with an electric mixer on medium speed until fluffy. Stir in 1 cup flour, ½ teaspoon lemon zest, and lemon extract, if desired. Press dough into an ungreased 8-inch pan, leveling surface. Bake 20 minutes.

2. Meanwhile, in same bowl, beat eggs with an electric mixer on medium speed until light and fluffy. In a small bowl, stir together 1¼ cups powdered sugar, remaining 2 tablespoons flour, and baking powder. Add to eggs and beat until blended. Stir in lemon juice and remaining zest.

3. Pour egg-sugar mixture over warm crust and return to oven. Bake 20 to 25 minutes, or until set. Remove pan to a rack and let cool completely in pan. To serve, sprinkle remaining 2 tablespoons powdered sugar on top and cut into 30 small bars. Store in refrigerator.

226 GRANOLA BARS

Prep: 10 minutes   Bake: 20 to 25 minutes   Makes: 30

These crisp, crunchy bars pack well and provide quick energy on the trail or the ski slope.

¾ cup whole wheat flour
½ teaspoon baking soda
½ teaspoon cinnamon
¼ teaspoon salt
¼ cup vegetable oil
½ cup firmly packed brown
    sugar

1 egg
½ teaspoon vanilla extract
1 cup rolled oats
1 cup corn or wheat flakes
½ cup raisins
¼ cup oat bran
2 tablespoons sesame seeds

1. Preheat oven to 350°F. Grease a 9 × 13-inch baking pan. In a small bowl, stir together flour, baking soda, cinnamon, and salt.

2. In a large bowl, beat oil, brown sugar, egg, and vanilla with an electric mixer on medium speed until fluffy and smooth, scraping down side of bowl frequently with a rubber spatula. Beat in flour mixture until soft dough forms.

3. Fold oatmeal, cornflakes, raisins, oat bran, and sesame seeds into soft dough. Spread dough in pan, leveling surface.

4. Bake 20 to 25 minutes, or until top is golden brown and a toothpick inserted in center comes out clean. Remove pan to a rack, cut into 30 bars, and let cool completely. Store in an airtight container.

227 PRALINE BARS

Prep: 10 minutes   Bake: 30 to 35 minutes   Makes: 16 to 20

1 cup plus 2 tablespoons flour
½ cup granulated sugar
1 stick (4 ounces) butter,
    softened
1 cup plus 2 tablespoons
    firmly packed light
    brown sugar

2 eggs
1 teaspoon vanilla extract
½ cup chopped pecans

1. Preheat oven to 375°F. In a small bowl, combine 1 cup flour with granulated sugar and butter. Stir until mixture resembles coarse meal. Press into bottom of an ungreased 8-inch square pan. Bake 15 minutes. Remove to a rack. Leave oven on.

2. In a medium bowl, beat together brown sugar, eggs, remaining 2 tablespoons flour, and vanilla. Stir in pecans. Pour over crust.

3. Return to oven and bake 15 to 20 minutes, or until filling is set. Remove pan to rack, cut into bars, and let cool completely in pan before serving.

228 PECAN BARS
Prep: 15 minutes   Bake: 40 to 45 minutes   Makes: 36

All the sweet Southern goodness of a pecan pie is packed into each of these little bar cookies. For best flavor, be sure your pecans are fresh. After opening a package, store the nuts in the freezer.

1 cup flour
1 stick (4 ounces) butter, softened, plus 1 tablespoon, melted
3 tablespoons powdered sugar
½ cup firmly packed dark brown sugar

1 cup dark or light corn syrup
3 eggs
1 tablespoon dark rum
1 teaspoon vanilla extract
¼ teaspoon salt
1½ cups chopped pecans

1. Preheat oven to 350°F. In a small bowl, combine flour, softened butter, and powdered sugar. Stir until mixture resembles coarse meal. Press into an ungreased 9-inch square pan. Bake 10 minutes, or until crust is lightly colored.

2. Meanwhile, in a medium bowl, beat together brown sugar, corn syrup, melted butter, eggs, rum, vanilla, and salt. Stir in pecans. Pour over partially baked crust.

3. Return to oven and bake 30 to 35 minutes, or until filling is set. Remove pan to a rack, cut into 36 bars, and let cool completely in pan before serving.

229 OATMEAL SHORTBREAD BARS
Prep: 5 minutes   Bake: 25 to 30 minutes   Makes: 25

1 stick (4 ounces) butter, softened
⅓ cup sugar

¾ cup flour
⅓ cup rolled oats
¼ teaspoon salt

1. Preheat oven to 325°F. Grease a 9-inch square pan.

2. In a medium bowl, beat butter and sugar with an electric mixer on medium speed until light and fluffy. Add flour, oatmeal, and salt and beat until blended. Press dough evenly over bottom of prepared pan.

3. Bake 25 to 30 minutes, until golden. Cut into bars while hot. Transfer to a rack and let cool in pan.

230 PUMPKIN BARS
Prep: 10 minutes   Bake: 25 to 30 minutes   Makes: 24

2 cups flour
2 teaspoons baking powder
2 teaspoons cinnamon
½ teaspoon grated nutmeg
½ teaspoon ground ginger
¼ teaspoon salt
1 cup firmly packed brown
    sugar

1 cup mashed cooked
    pumpkin
1 stick (4 ounces) butter,
    softened
1 egg
2 teaspoons vanilla extract
½ cup chopped walnuts
½ cup raisins

1. Preheat oven to 350°F. Grease a 9 × 13-inch baking pan. In a medium bowl, stir together flour, baking powder, cinnamon, nutmeg, ginger, and salt.

2. In a large bowl, beat brown sugar, pumpkin, butter, egg, and vanilla with an electric mixer on medium speed until smooth. Add flour mixture and beat on low speed just until batter is smooth, scraping down side of bowl frequently with a rubber spatula. Fold in nuts and raisins. Turn batter into prepared pan, leveling surface.

3. Bake 25 to 30 minutes, or until top is golden brown and a toothpick inserted in center comes out clean. Remove pan to a rack, cut into 24 bars, and let cool completely. Store in an airtight container or wrap well and refrigerate.

---

231 TREASURE BARS
Prep: 10 minutes   Bake: 37 to 45 minutes   Makes: 25

1 cup flour
½ cup powdered sugar
1 stick (4 ounces) butter,
    softened
½ teaspoon salt
½ cup light corn syrup

½ cup firmly packed dark
    brown sugar
¼ cup peanut butter
2 eggs
1 teaspoon vanilla extract
¾ cup semisweet chocolate
    chips

1. Preheat oven to 350°F. In a large bowl, beat flour, powdered sugar, butter, and ¼ teaspoon salt with an electric mixer on medium speed until blended. Press into an ungreased 9-inch square pan, leveling surface. Bake 12 to 15 minutes, until edges brown.

2. Meanwhile, in a medium bowl, beat corn syrup, brown sugar, peanut butter, eggs, ¼ teaspoon salt, and vanilla with electric mixer on medium speed until well blended.

3. Pour over warm crust, sprinkle with chocolate chips, and return to oven. Bake 25 to 30 minutes, or until filling is set and lightly browned. Remove pan to a rack and let cool completely before cutting into 25 bars.

232 PEPPERMINT SQUARES

Prep: 10 minutes   Bake: 15 to 20 minutes   Makes: 16

Thin chocolate-covered mints form the top layer of these aromatic cookies. Be sure to store them in their own tin, as the mint flavor will be picked up by more delicately flavored cookies.

4 tablespoons butter, softened	1 cup flour
¼ cup firmly packed brown sugar	16 (1½-inch square) thin chocolate-covered mints
1 teaspoon vanilla extract	

1. Preheat oven to 350°F. Grease an 8-inch square pan.

2. In a small bowl, beat butter, brown sugar, and vanilla with an electric mixer on medium speed until fluffy. On low speed, beat in flour until a crumbly dough forms, scraping down side of bowl frequently with a rubber spatula. Turn into prepared pan. With floured fingers, firmly pat crumbly mixture over bottom in an even layer.

3. Bake 15 to 20 minutes, or until top is golden brown and a toothpick inserted in center comes out clean. Remove pan to a rack. Immediately arrange mints on top of hot baked crust. Set aside 10 minutes for chocolate-covered mints to melt.

4. If desired, make a feathered design by pulling the tip of a knife crosswise through chocolate, reversing direction every other line. Cut into 16 squares and let cool completely. Store in an airtight container or wrap well and refrigerate.

Chapter 10

American Classics

Cookies came to America with the earliest colonists. The word itself is probably Dutch in origin, from *koekje*, the diminutive of *koek*, or cake. Because refined sugar was expensive and not always readily available, many of the first American cookies were sweetened with honey or molasses. As soon as sugar became more commonplace, however, traditional Old World recipes were used to reproduce the cookies remembered from homes across the sea. Many early American cookies were called jumbles. There doesn't seem to be any universal ingredient or characteristic for a jumble; some were simple sugar cookies, while others were quite spicy.

The cookies in this chapter are in most cases early twentieth-century recipes that were handed down through recent generations. They are the cookies most likely to be found in American cookie jars today and those we all remember hoping for in elementary school lunch bags a few decades past. They are not the holiday cookies that require special, sometimes expensive, ingredients, but those that can be thrown together after work from staple ingredients that are in almost everyone's cupboard.

A look at the original versions of these recipes reminded us of the changes that have occurred in American recipes in the past few years. Most of the recipes were just lists of ingredients, because it was assumed that everyone already knew how to put them together. Those that did have directions usually started with a thorough "creaming" of the butter and sugar. Although we still begin our cookie preparation by beating the softened butter and the sugar together until air has been incorporated and the dough is light and creamy, perhaps even cream colored, we no longer use the verb "to cream," because many cooks today do not recognize it.

Testing these recipes brought back memories of coming home from school to the aroma of fresh-baked cookies and of our own first cookie-baking experiences. Turn to this chapter to rediscover the taste of your childhood favorites and to create new memories for your own family.

233   LADY BALTIMORE COOKIES
Prep: 10 minutes   Bake: 10 minutes   Stand: 2 hours
Makes: about 36

Inspired by the filling of the famous Lady Baltimore cake, these sweet meringue cookies have a crisp white exterior and a chewy fruit and nut center.

3 **egg whites, at room temperature**	¼ **cup chopped pecans**
½ **teaspoon cream of tartar**	¼ **cup chopped raisins**
¼ **teaspoon salt**	¼ **cup chopped candied cherries**
¾ **cup sugar**	1 **tablespoon brandy**

1. Preheat oven to 275°F. In a medium bowl, beat egg whites, cream of tartar, and salt with an electric mixer on high speed until frothy. Very slowly beat in sugar, a little at a time. Continue to beat until whites are very stiff. Fold in pecans, raisins, cherries, and brandy.

2. Drop by heaping teaspoonfuls 2 inches apart onto parchment- or foil-lined cookie sheets. Bake 10 minutes. Turn off oven and leave cookies in unopened oven for 2 hours. Remove cookies from sheets and store in a tightly covered container.

234   BACHELOR BUTTONS
Prep: 10 minutes   Bake: 12 to 15 minutes   Makes: about 48

We don't know whether this old-fashioned recipe was named for its flowerlike appearance or because the cookies were known to attract eligible young men.

1½ **sticks (6 ounces) butter, softened**	1 **teaspoon baking powder**
1 **cup firmly packed brown sugar**	½ **teaspoon baking soda**
	½ **teaspoon cinnamon**
1 **egg**	¼ **teaspoon ground ginger**
½ **teaspoon vanilla extract**	¼ **teaspoon salt**
2 **cups flour**	24 **red candied cherries, halved**

1. Preheat oven to 350°F. In a large bowl, beat butter and brown sugar with an electric mixer on medium speed until well blended. Beat in egg and vanilla until light and fluffy.

2. Add flour mixed with baking powder, baking soda, cinnamon, ginger, and salt and beat until dough is smooth, scraping down side of bowl frequently with a rubber spatula.

3. Drop by heaping teaspoonfuls 2 inches apart onto lightly greased cookie sheets. Press a cherry half into center of each ball of dough. Bake 12 to 15 minutes, or until golden brown. Let cookies cool 2 minutes on sheets, then remove to racks and let cool completely. Store in a tightly covered container.

235 BLACK AND WHITES

Prep: 10 minutes   Bake: 18 to 20 minutes   Makes: about 18

1 **egg**	1 **teaspoon baking powder**
¾ **cup sugar**	¼ **teaspoon baking soda**
⅓ **cup melted butter**	¼ **teaspoon salt**
2 **teaspoons vanilla extract**	**Black and White Frosting**
½ **cup buttermilk**	**(recipe follows)**
1¾ **cups cake flour**	

1. Preheat oven to 350°F. Separate egg. Place white in a small bowl and beat with an electric mixer on high speed until soft peaks form. Gradually add ¼ cup sugar, beating until stiff peaks form when beaters are raised.

2. In a large bowl, with same beaters, beat remaining ½ cup sugar, melted butter, egg yolk, and vanilla with electric mixer on medium speed until well blended. Beat in buttermilk. Add cake flour mixed with baking powder, baking soda, and salt and beat until a stiff batter forms. With a wire whisk, gently fold in beaten egg white.

3. Drop by heaping measuring tablespoonfuls 3 inches apart onto lightly greased cookie sheets. Bake 18 to 20 minutes, or until edges are golden brown. Let cookies cool 2 minutes on sheets, then remove to racks to cool completely.

4. Meanwhile prepare frosting. Frost half of bottom flat surface of cooled cookies with white frosting and half with chocolate frosting. Set aside until surface of frosting has dried, at least 1 hour. Store between layers of wax paper in a tightly covered container.

BLACK AND WHITE FROSTING

2 **cups powdered sugar**	⅛ **teaspoon salt**
¼ **cup solid vegetable**	½ **ounce (½ square)**
shortening	**unsweetened chocolate,**
3 **to 4 tablespoons milk**	**melted**
½ **teaspoon vanilla extract**	

1. Reserve 2 tablespoons powdered sugar. In a medium bowl, beat remaining powdered sugar, shortening, 3 tablespoons milk, vanilla, and salt until smooth. Add remaining milk, if necessary, to make white frosting manageable.

2. Remove half of frosting to a small bowl. With a fork, stir in remaining powdered sugar and melted chocolate until chocolate frosting is smooth and well blended.

236 BENNE SEED WAFERS
Prep: 10 minutes   Bake: 8 to 10 minutes   Makes: about 50

½ cup sesame seeds
1 stick (4 ounces) butter, softened
½ cup firmly packed brown sugar

1 teaspoon vanilla extract
¾ cup flour
¼ teaspoon baking soda
⅛ teaspoon salt

1. Preheat oven to 350°F. Spread out sesame seeds on a small baking sheet. Bake until they just start to turn golden, 3 to 5 minutes. Transfer from baking sheet to a large bowl immediately.

2. Add butter, brown sugar, and vanilla to sesame seeds and beat with an electric mixer on medium speed until light and fluffy. Beat in flour mixed with baking soda and salt until dough is smooth, scraping down side of bowl frequently with a rubber spatula.

3. Drop by measuring teaspoonfuls 2 inches apart onto lightly greased cookie sheets. Bake 8 to 10 minutes, or until edges are golden brown. Let cookies cool 2 minutes on sheets, then remove to racks and let cool completely. Store in a tightly covered container.

237 GINGERSNAPS
Prep: 10 minutes   Bake: 12 to 15 minutes   Makes: about 42

A tiny drop of water on each cookie just before baking makes the difference between a shiny and a dull sugar-crinkled top.

1½ sticks (6 ounces) butter, softened
1⅓ cups sugar
1 egg
¼ cup light molasses
2 cups flour

2 teaspoons ground ginger
1 teaspoon baking soda
1 teaspoon cinnamon
¼ teaspoon ground cloves
¼ teaspoon salt

1. Preheat oven to 350°F. In a large bowl, beat butter and 1 cup sugar with an electric mixer on medium speed until well blended. Beat in egg and molasses until light and fluffy.

2. Beat in flour mixed with ginger, baking soda, cinnamon, cloves, and salt until dough is smooth, scraping down side of bowl frequently with a rubber spatula.

3. Divide dough into 1-inch balls. Roll balls in remaining ⅓ cup sugar and place 2½ inches apart on greased baking sheets (snaps will spread a lot). With fingertip, place a drop of water on top of each cookie; do not press balls down.

4. Bake 12 to 15 minutes, or until flattened and crinkled. Let cookies cool 2 minutes on sheets, then remove to racks to cool completely. Store in a tightly covered container.

238 RASPBERRY TEA CAKES

Prep: 10 minutes   Chill: 2 hours   Bake: 10 to 12 minutes
Makes: about 36

1 stick (4 ounces) butter,
    softened
½ cup sugar
1 egg
1 teaspoon vanilla extract

1¼ cups flour
⅛ teaspoon salt
¼ cup finely chopped pecans
¼ cup seedless red raspberry
    jam

1. In a medium bowl, beat butter and sugar with an electric mixer on medium speed until well blended. Beat in egg and vanilla until light and fluffy.

2. Add flour and salt and beat on low speed until dough is smooth, scraping down side of bowl frequently with a rubber spatula. Wrap and refrigerate dough 2 to 3 hours, until firm.

3. Preheat oven to 350°F. Using about 1 measuring teaspoonful in each, press dough into miniature muffin pan cups to cover bottoms and up sides. In a small bowl, crumble remaining dough and mix with pecans. Divide jam into dough-lined cups, using a slightly rounded measuring ¼ teaspoon in each. Sprinkle pecan mixture over top.

4. Bake 10 to 12 minutes, or until crust is golden brown and jam is bubbly. Let cool 5 minutes in pans, then remove to racks and let cool completely. Store in a tightly covered container.

---

239 COCONUT MACAROONS

Prep: 10 minutes   Bake: 8 to 10 minutes   Makes: about 60

Sweetened condensed milk has been a real time saver for cooks ever since its development over a hundred years ago.

2 (7-ounce) packages flaked
    coconut
1 (14-ounce) can sweetened
    condensed milk (*not*
    evaporated milk)

2 teaspoons vanilla extract
1½ teaspoons almond extract

1. Preheat oven to 350°F. In a large bowl, combine coconut, sweetened condensed milk, vanilla, and almond extract. Mix until well blended.

2. Drop by heaping teaspoonfuls 2 inches apart onto aluminum foil–lined cookie sheets.

3. Bake 8 to 10 minutes, or until lightly browned around edges. Immediately remove to racks and let cool completely. Store loosely covered at room temperature.

Recipe reprinted courtesy of *Eagle Brand Sweetened Condensed Milk*.

240   DREAM BARS
Prep: 15 minutes   Bake: 27 to 35 minutes   Makes: 20

There are dozens of variations of this cookie, which was a favorite during the 1940s and '50s.

1   stick (4 ounces) butter, softened
¼   cup granulated sugar
1   cup flour
½   teaspoon cinnamon
1   egg
¼   cup firmly packed brown sugar
1½   teaspoons cornstarch
¼   teaspoon baking powder
⅛   teaspoon salt
½   cup coarsely chopped walnuts
½   cup flaked coconut

1. Preheat oven to 350°F. Generously grease a 9-inch square pan.

2. In a medium bowl, beat butter and granulated sugar with an electric mixer on medium speed until fluffy. Stir in flour and cinnamon until a soft dough forms.

3. Turn dough into prepared pan. With floured fingers, pat dough gently to make an even crust. Bake 12 to 15 minutes, or until center is no longer puffed.

4. In same bowl, beat together egg, brown sugar, cornstarch, baking powder, and salt with an electric mixer on medium speed until smooth. Fold in nuts and coconut. Spread mixture evenly over partially baked crust and return to oven.

5. Bake 15 to 20 minutes, or until top is set and lightly browned. Remove pan to a rack, cut into 20 bars, and let cool completely. Store, covered, in refrigerator.

241   FAMOUS OATMEAL COOKIES
Prep: 10 minutes   Bake: 12 to 15 minutes   Makes: about 60

This recipe appeared on the Quaker Oats box for many years and is part of many families' collections of most-used recipes.

¾   cup solid vegetable shortening
1   cup firmly packed brown sugar
½   cup granulated sugar
1   egg
1   teaspoon vanilla extract
1   cup flour
1   teaspoon salt (optional)
½   teaspoon baking soda
3   cups rolled oats

1. Preheat oven to 350°F. In a large bowl, beat shortening, brown sugar, granulated sugar, egg, ¼ cup water, and vanilla with an electric mixer on medium speed until creamy.

2. Beat in flour mixed with salt and baking soda until dough is smooth, scraping down side of bowl frequently with a rubber spatula. Fold in oatmeal. Drop by heaping teaspoonfuls 2 inches apart onto ungreased cookie sheets.

3. Bake 12 to 15 minutes, or until golden brown. Let cookies cool 2 minutes on sheets, then remove to racks and let cool completely. Store in a tightly covered container.

Recipe reprinted courtesy of *Quaker Oats*.

---

242   GRAHAM CRACKERS
Prep: 20 minutes   Bake: 15 to 20 minutes   Makes: 64

Early in the nineteenth century, the Reverend Sylvester Graham advocated the use of whole wheat flour for its nutritional value. His specially formulated whole wheat flour became known as graham flour, and these classic all-American cookies were one of the most popular uses for it.

2½ cups whole wheat flour	¼ teaspoon salt
1½ cups all-purpose flour	⅔ cup solid vegetable
¼ cup sugar	shortening,
2 teaspoons baking powder	melted
2 teaspoons cinnamon	½ cup honey
½ teaspoon grated nutmeg	½ cup apple juice or cider

1. Preheat oven to 350°F. In a medium bowl, combine whole wheat flour, all-purpose flour, sugar, baking powder, cinnamon, nutmeg, and salt. In a small bowl, combine melted shortening, honey, and apple juice. Stir to mix well. Make a well in center of flour mixture; pour honey mixture into well. With a fork, stir mixture until a stiff dough forms. Knead dough into a ball; divide into 4 balls and set aside.

2. On lightly greased cookie sheets, roll out each ball of dough to make a 10-inch square. With a knife or pastry wheel, cut each dough square into sixteen 2½-inch square crackers. With tines of a fork, pierce each cracker 3 times. (See Note.)

3. Bake 15 minutes, or until edges begin to brown. Carefully remove crisp outer crackers to rack. Separate 4 inner crackers and any others that don't seem crisp. Return to oven 5 minutes longer, then remove to racks and let cool completely. Store in a tightly covered container.

   NOTE: *If you do not have 4 cookie sheets, roll out dough on pieces of aluminum foil and bake on the cookie sheets you have. When one batch of crackers is completely baked, remove to a cooling rack and place another piece of unbaked dough on foil onto cookie sheet. Repeat until all have been baked.*

243 OATMEAL RAISIN COOKIES
Prep: 10 minutes   Bake: 10 to 12 minutes   Makes: about 36

These are one of our favorite cookies to send to children away at school or summer camp.

½ cup firmly packed brown sugar	1½ cups flour
1 stick (4 ounces) butter, softened	½ teaspoon baking soda
	¼ teaspoon salt
1 egg	1 cup rolled oats
¼ cup light molasses	½ cup raisins

1. Preheat oven to 350°F. In a large bowl, beat brown sugar, butter, egg, and molasses with an electric mixer on medium speed until well blended.

2. Beat in flour mixed with baking soda and salt until dough is smooth, scraping down side of bowl frequently with a rubber spatula. Fold in oatmeal and raisins.

3. Drop dough by heaping teaspoonfuls 2 inches apart onto lightly greased cookie sheets. Bake 10 to 12 minutes, or until golden brown. Let cookies cool 2 minutes on sheets, then remove to racks and let cool completely. Store in a tightly covered container.

244 PEANUT BUTTER KISS COOKIES
Prep: 10 minutes   Bake: 10 to 12 minutes   Makes: about 50

1 cup chunky peanut butter	2½ cups flour
¾ cup firmly packed brown sugar	1 teaspoon baking soda
	¼ teaspoon salt
1 stick (4 ounces) butter, softened	¼ cup unsalted peanuts, finely chopped
2 eggs	1 (9-ounce) package milk chocolate kisses
1 teaspoon vanilla extract	

1. Preheat oven to 350°F. In a large bowl, beat peanut butter, brown sugar, and butter with an electric mixer on medium speed until light and fluffy. Beat in eggs and vanilla until well blended.

2. Mix flour, baking soda, and salt and beat in until dough is smooth, scraping down side of bowl frequently with a rubber spatula.

3. Drop by heaping teaspoonfuls 2 inches apart onto lightly greased cookie sheets. Sprinkle chopped peanuts onto tops of cookies; press dough to flatten slightly.

4. Bake 8 minutes. Meanwhile, remove foil wrappers from kisses. Remove cookies from oven; leave oven on. Carefully press a kiss pointed side up into the center of each cookie. Return to oven and bake 2 to 4 minutes longer, or until golden brown. Let cookies cool 2 minutes on sheets, then remove to racks and let cool completely. Store in a tightly covered container.

245 HERMITS
Prep: 10 minutes   Bake: 12 to 15 minutes   Makes: about 48

We have added dried cherries instead of maraschino cherries to this old family recipe. We recommend black walnuts as a first choice here, because they add an intensely nutty flavor (see Mail Order Sources on page 4). These pack very well, which makes them a good choice for lunch boxes or for mailing to summer camp or college.

1 stick (4 ounces) butter, softened	1 cup raisins
¼ cup sugar	½ cup dried cherries
1 egg	½ cup dried apples, chopped
¼ cup orange juice	½ cup pitted dates, chopped
1½ cups flour	½ cup walnuts, preferably black walnuts, coarsely chopped
½ teaspoon baking soda	
½ teaspoon cinnamon	Glaze (optional; recipe follows)
¼ teaspoon salt	

1. Preheat oven to 350°F. In a large bowl, beat butter and sugar with an electric mixer on medium speed until well blended. Beat in egg and orange juice until light and fluffy.

2. Beat in flour mixed with baking soda, cinnamon, and salt on low speed until well blended, scraping down side of bowl frequently with a rubber spatula. Stir in raisins, cherries, apples, dates, and walnuts.

3. Drop by heaping teaspoonfuls 2 inches apart onto lightly greased cookie sheets. Bake 12 to 15 minutes, or until golden brown. Let cookies cool 2 minutes on sheets, then remove to racks and let cool completely.

4. If desired, prepare glaze and drizzle over cooled cookies. Let dry completely and store in a tightly covered container.

GLAZE

In a small bowl, stir together ⅓ cup powdered sugar and 1½ to 2 teaspoons orange juice to make a pourable glaze.

246 GRANDMA LAMB'S MOLASSES COOKIES
Prep: 10 minutes   Bake: 15 to 18 minutes   Makes: about 32

Joanne learned to make these cookies from her grandmother's recipe when she first started baking. They are not too sweet and were often part of a hearty farm breakfast. These are best served freshly baked.

⅔ cup solid vegetable shortening	1 teaspoon baking soda
⅓ cup sugar	1 teaspoon ground ginger
1 egg	1 teaspoon cinnamon
¾ cup light molasses	¼ teaspoon ground cloves
½ cup buttermilk	¼ teaspoon salt
2⅓ cups flour	½ cup chopped raisins

1. Preheat oven to 350°F. In a large bowl, beat shortening, sugar, and egg with an electric mixer on medium speed until well blended. Beat in molasses and buttermilk, then flour mixed with baking soda, ginger, cinnamon, cloves, and salt until a soft dough forms. Fold in raisins.

2. Drop by heaping measuring tablespoonfuls 3 inches apart onto lightly greased cookie sheets. Bake 15 to 18 minutes, or until edges are golden brown. Let cookies cool 2 minutes on sheets, then remove to racks to cool completely. Store in a tightly covered container.

247 SUGAR JUMBLES
Prep: 10 minutes   Chill: 30 minutes   Bake: 10 to 12 minutes
Makes: about 48

In Colonial days many simple cookies were called jumbles. This soft sugar cookie dough is easy to assemble and delightfully buttery.

¾ cup granulated sugar	1½ cups flour
1 stick (4 ounces) butter, softened	½ teaspoon baking powder
¼ cup sour cream	⅛ teaspoon salt
1½ teaspoons vanilla extract	Colored crystal sugar or granulated sugar

1. In a medium bowl, beat granulated sugar and butter with an electric mixer on medium speed until well blended. Beat in sour cream and vanilla until light and fluffy.

2. On low speed, beat in flour mixed with baking powder and salt until dough is smooth, scraping down side of bowl frequently with a rubber spatula. Wrap dough and refrigerate 30 minutes.

3. Preheat oven to 350°F. Form dough into 1-inch balls. Place 2 inches apart on lightly greased cookie sheets. With bottom of a glass dipped into colored or granulated sugar, press each ball of dough to flatten slightly.

4. Bake 10 to 12 minutes, or until edges are golden brown. Let cookies cool 2 minutes on sheets, then remove to wire racks and let cool completely. Store in a tightly covered container.

---

248 ORIGINAL TOLL HOUSE COOKIES
Prep: 10 minutes Bake: 9 to 11 minutes Makes: about 60

In the 1930s, Ruth Wakefield, proprietor of the Toll House Inn near Whitman, Massachusetts, was experimenting with a popular Colonial cookie—The Butter Drop Do. She chopped up a bar of Nestlé's semisweet chocolate into tiny bits and added them to the cookie dough, creating the first Toll House Cookie. With Mrs. Wakefield's permission, Nestlé put the recipe for her cookies right on the wrapper of its semisweet chocolate bar. Soon after, Nestlé began producing semisweet chocolate morsels, or chips, and the cookies made from the recipe that appears on the back of each bag of Nestlé Toll House morsels have since become an American favorite.

2¼ cups flour	1 teaspoon vanilla extract
1 teaspoon baking soda	2 eggs
1 teaspoon salt	12 ounces (2 cups) Nestlé Toll
2 sticks (8 ounces) butter,	House semisweet
softened	chocolate morsels
¾ cup granulated sugar	1 cup chopped nuts
¾ cup firmly packed brown	
sugar	

1. Preheat oven to 375°F. In a small bowl, combine flour, baking soda, and salt. In a large bowl, combine butter, granulated sugar, brown sugar, and vanilla; beat until creamy. Add eggs, one at a time, beating well after each addition. Gradually beat in dry ingredients. Stir in chocolate morsels and nuts.

2. Drop by rounded measuring tablespoonfuls 2 inches apart onto ungreased cookie sheets. Bake 9 to 11 minutes, or until golden brown. Let cookies cool 2 minutes on sheets, then remove to racks and let cool completely. Store in a tightly covered container.

Recipe reprinted courtesy of *Nestlé USA, Inc.*

249 SHORTENIN' BREAD

Prep: 20 minutes   Bake: 10 to 12 minutes   Makes: about 20

Nineteenth-century cooks often just added sugar to their pastry recipe to make these flaky cookies. We have substituted a mixture of butter and vegetable shortening for the lard traditionally used.

1½ cups flour
¼ cup sugar
½ teaspoon salt
4 tablespoons cold unsalted butter

2 tablespoons solid vegetable shortening
3 to 4 tablespoons cold water
1 tablespoon coarse sugar or crushed sugar cubes

1. Preheat oven to 350°F. In a medium bowl, stir together flour, sugar, and salt. With a pastry blender or 2 knives, cut in butter and shortening until mixture resembles coarse crumbs. With a fork, gradually stir in 3 tablespoons water until mixture forms a ball of dough. Add a little more water, if necessary, to make dough manageable.

2. Shape dough into a flattened ball. Between pieces of wax paper, roll out dough ¼ inch thick. Cut out rounds with a 2-inch cookie cutter. Reroll scraps to make additional cookies. Sprinkle coarse sugar or crushed sugar cubes on top.

3. Place dough rounds 2 inches apart on lightly greased cookie sheets. Bake 10 to 12 minutes, or until edges are golden brown. Let cookies cool 2 minutes on sheets, then remove to racks and let cool completely. Store in a tightly covered container.

250 GRANDMA LEESE'S SUGAR COOKIES

Prep: 10 minutes   Bake: 18 to 20 minutes   Makes: about 18

Joanne remembers that her grandmother always had a tin of these giant cookies on top of her refrigerator awaiting the family's Saturday visit. She usually made them with the chicken fat she had saved from preparing a large pot of chicken soup. The chicken fat gave the cookies a rich flavor and a beautiful golden color. Today, Joanne usually makes them with melted vegetable shortening. These are best when freshly baked.

1 cup granulated sugar
⅓ cup melted vegetable shortening, chicken fat, or vegetable oil
1 egg
2 teaspoons vanilla extract

½ cup milk
1¾ cups flour
1 teaspoon baking powder
¼ teaspoon salt
¼ cup raisins (optional)
   Powdered sugar

1. Preheat oven to 350°F. In a large bowl, beat granulated sugar, shortening, egg, and vanilla with an electric mixer on medium speed until well blended. Beat in milk, then flour mixed with baking powder and salt until a stiff dough forms. Stir in raisins if you feel like adding them.

2. Drop by heaping measuring tablespoonfuls 3 inches apart onto lightly greased cookie sheets. Bake 18 to 20 minutes, or until edges are golden brown. Let cookies cool 2 minutes on sheets, then remove to racks to cool completely. Store in a tightly covered container. Dust with powdered sugar before serving.

---

251 SNICKERDOODLES
Prep: 10 minutes   Bake: 8 to 10 minutes   Makes: about 36

Although the name is just a nineteenth-century nonsense word, and the recipe varies slightly from home to home, the crinkly cinnamon coating distinguishes these traditional New England cookies.

¾ cup sugar	1⅓ cups flour
1 stick (4 ounces) butter, softened	1 teaspoon baking powder
	¼ teaspoon salt
1 egg	1 teaspoon cinnamon
½ teaspoon vanilla extract	

1. Preheat oven to 350°F. Reserve 1 tablespoon sugar. In a large bowl, beat remaining sugar and butter with an electric mixer on medium speed until well blended. Beat in egg and vanilla until light and fluffy.

2. Add flour mixed with baking powder and salt and beat on low speed until a stiff dough forms, scraping down side of bowl frequently with a rubber spatula. Form dough into 1-inch balls.

3. In a small bowl, stir together reserved 1 tablespoon sugar with cinnamon to make cinnamon sugar. Roll balls in cinnamon sugar and place 2 inches apart on lightly greased baking sheets.

4. Bake cookies 8 to 10 minutes, or until flattened and firm in center. Let cookies cool 2 minutes on sheets, then remove to racks and let cool completely. Store in a tightly covered container.

Chapter 11

International Favorites

Each wave of immigrants that came to America brought with them the cookie traditions of their homeland. These are the unique cookies discovered in ethnic bakeries and the secret family recipes served to special guests. They are a reminder of the rich diversity of our culture and of the gradual assimilation of each ethnic group's food traditions into the national culture. While some of these cookies are still unusual, most are already being enjoyed in many households across the country.

Because the recipes in this chapter come from a variety of traditions, there are techniques used here that you won't find elsewhere in the book. Several of the cookies require special top-of-the-stove "irons" for baking; others are fried. These techniques might have originally allowed home cooks to produce sweet treats in a kitchen without an oven. Even after baking moved from the communal village oven to an oven in every home, the unique flavor of these cookies kept them on the cookie menu of their culture. When preparing fried cookies, it is important to use sufficient melted shortening or oil to cover the cookies without allowing them to touch the bottom of the pan. The frying temperature should be checked with a deep-fat thermometer before the cookies are placed in the fat and periodically during the frying period. Although it is time consuming, it is important to fry only as many cookies at a time as the pan can hold without their touching each other. All fried cookies should, of course, be well drained before serving.

It was sometimes hard to know whether to put many of these cookies here or in the celebrations chapter, because we found that many people only get around to making their family's traditional Old World cookies for holidays and celebrations. In most cases we decided on the basis of whether they were celebration cookies or year-round cookies in their original setting. We hope this chapter will encourage you to rediscover your favorite traditional cookies and to make them often.

252 ALMOND BISCOTTI

Prep: 15 minutes   Bake: 40 to 42 minutes   Makes: 24

Biscotti are crisp Italian twice-baked cookies, which are particularly good with coffee or tea.

⅔ cup blanched almonds
2 eggs
1 teaspoon almond extract
⅔ cup sugar

1½ cups cake flour
1 teaspoon baking powder
¼ teaspoon salt

1. Preheat oven to 350°F. Spread almonds out on a small baking sheet. Place in oven and toast 6 to 8 minutes, or until golden. Remove and let cool; coarsely chop toasted almonds.

2. In a medium bowl, beat eggs with an electric mixer on high speed until fluffy. Gradually beat in almond extract and sugar until mixture is thick and lemon colored, scraping down side of bowl frequently. With a rubber spatula, fold in cake flour mixed with baking powder and salt just until thoroughly combined. Fold in chopped toasted almonds.

3. Grease a 10 × 4-inch strip down center of 2 cookie sheets. Spoon half of almond mixture down center of each cookie sheet to make a 3 × 10-inch log. Bake 30 minutes. Remove from oven; leave oven on.

4. Let cookies cool on sheets 3 to 5 minutes, or just until cool enough to handle. With a serrated knife, cut each log diagonally into 12 slices. Place slices, flat sides down, on cookie sheets and return to oven 5 minutes. Turn slices over and bake 5 to 7 minutes longer, or until golden on both sides. Remove to racks and let cool completely. Store in a tightly covered container.

253 CHOCOLATE BISCOTTI

Prep: 10 minutes   Bake: 40 to 42 minutes   Makes: 24

2 eggs
1 teaspoon vanilla extract
⅔ cup sugar
1¼ cups cake flour
⅓ cup unsweetened cocoa
powder

1 teaspoon baking powder
¼ teaspoon salt
¼ cup miniature chocolate
chips
⅓ cup pine nuts (pignoli)

1. Preheat oven to 350°F. In a medium bowl, beat eggs with an electric mixer on high speed until fluffy. Gradually beat in vanilla and sugar until mixture is thick and lemon colored, scraping down side of bowl frequently with a rubber spatula.

2. With a wire whisk, fold in cake flour mixed with cocoa powder, baking powder, and salt just until thoroughly combined. Fold in chocolate chips and pine nuts.

3. Grease a 10 × 4-inch strip down center of 2 cookie sheets. Spoon half of chocolate mixture down center of each cookie sheet to make a 3 × 10-inch log. Bake 30 minutes. Remove from oven; leave oven on.

4. Let logs cool on sheets 3 to 5 minutes, or just until cool enough to handle. With a serrated knife, cut each log diagonally into 12 slices. Place slices, flat sides down, on cookie sheets and return to oven. Bake 5 minutes. Turn slices over and bake 5 to 7 minutes longer, or until crisp on both sides. Remove to racks and let cool completely. Store in a tightly covered container.

---

254 PISTACHIO BISCOTTI
Prep: 10 minutes   Bake: 40 to 42 minutes   Makes: 32

2 eggs
1 teaspoon almond extract
1 teaspoon vanilla extract
½ cup sugar
1¾ cups cake flour

1 teaspoon baking powder
¼ teaspoon salt
⅔ cup shelled pistachio nuts
3 ounces semisweet chocolate, melted

1. Preheat oven to 350°F. In a medium bowl, beat eggs with an electric mixer on high speed until fluffy. Gradually beat in almond extract, vanilla, and sugar until mixture is thick and lemon colored, scraping down side of bowl frequently with a rubber spatula.

2. With a wire whisk, fold in cake flour mixed with baking powder and salt just until thoroughly combined. Fold in pistachios.

3. Grease a 10 × 4-inch strip down center of 2 cookie sheets. Spoon half of pistachio mixture down center of each cookie sheet to make a 3 × 10-inch log. Bake 30 minutes. Remove from oven; leave oven on.

4. Let logs cool on sheets 5 minutes, or until cool enough to handle. With a serrated knife, cut each log diagonally into 16 slices. Place slices, flat sides down, on cookie sheets and return to oven. Bake 5 minutes. Turn slices over and bake 5 to 7 minutes longer, or until golden on both sides. Remove to racks and let stand until cool enough to handle. Spread melted chocolate over one end of biscotti and let cool completely. Store in a tightly covered container.

255   AMARETTI
Prep: 10 minutes   Bake: 30 minutes   Stand: 2 hours
Makes: about 28

European versions of these cookies are made partially of bitter almonds, which lend a more intense almond flavor and balance the sweetness of the sugar. We use almond extract instead to heighten the sensation.

2 egg whites	1 teaspoon almond extract
⅔ cup sugar	¼ teaspoon baking powder
1 cup ground blanched almonds	¼ teaspoon salt

1. Preheat oven to 250°F. Lightly grease 2 cookie sheets. In a medium bowl, beat egg whites with an electric mixer on medium speed until fluffy. Gradually beat in sugar and continue beating until mixture is stiff, scraping down side of bowl frequently with a rubber spatula.

2. Fold in almonds, almond extract, baking powder, and salt. Drop by heaping teaspoonfuls 2 inches apart onto prepared cookie sheets.

3. Bake 30 minutes. Turn off heat and leave amaretti in unopened oven 2 hours, or until crisp. Remove from sheets and store in a tightly covered container.

256   GERMAN PRETZEL COOKIES
Prep: 10 minutes   Bake: 10 to 12 minutes   Makes: 24

1 raw egg	2 hard-boiled egg yolks
½ cup sugar	1 teaspoon vanilla extract
1½ sticks (6 ounces) butter, softened	2 cups flour
	Colored sugar

1. Separate egg; set aside white. In a medium bowl, beat sugar, butter, and hard-boiled egg yolks with an electric mixer on medium speed until smooth. Add raw egg yolk and vanilla and beat until light and fluffy.

2. Gradually add flour and beat on low speed until dough is smooth, scraping down side of bowl frequently with a rubber spatula.

3. Preheat oven to 350°F. Make 24 ropes 7 inches long from dough, using about 1 heaping measuring teaspoon dough for each. Shape ropes into pretzels (see Note below) on lightly greased cookie sheets. Lightly beat reserved egg white; brush over pretzels. Sprinkle with colored sugar.

4. Bake 10 to 12 minutes, or until golden brown. Let cookies cool 2 minutes on sheets, then remove to racks and let cool completely. Store in a tightly covered container.

NOTE: *To form pretzels, place dough rope on a flat work surface in a U shape, like a horseshoe, with ends toward you. Lift ends, twist, and turn back toward bend of U. Spread ends apart and press onto dough about ¼ inch on either side of bend.*

257 CHOCOLATE CHOPSTICKS

Prep: 15 minutes Chill: 8 minutes Bake: 8 to 10 minutes
Makes: 96

We tried to duplicate the matchstick-thin, chocolate-tipped cookie sticks imported from Japan. Although these are not quite as delicate, we think they are just as delicious.

½ cup sugar	⅛ teaspoon salt
4 tablespoons butter, softened	¼ cup milk
1 egg	½ teaspoon vanilla extract
2½ cups flour	6 ounces semisweet chocolate
½ teaspoon baking powder	chips (1 cup), melted

1. In a large bowl, beat sugar and butter with an electric mixer on medium speed until well blended. Beat in egg until light and fluffy.

2. Mix flour, baking powder, and salt and add alternately with milk and vanilla, beating on low speed, until dough is smooth; scrape down side of bowl frequently with a rubber spatula.

3. Divide dough into 2 pieces. Between pieces of wax paper, roll out each piece into a 12-inch square. Still on wax paper, with a long knife, cut each dough square into 48 sticks ¼ × 12 inches. Lift dough squares onto a cookie sheet and place in the freezer 8 to 10 minutes, or until firm enough to remove from wax paper.

4. Preheat oven to 350°F. One at a time, slide chopsticks off wax paper onto lightly greased cookie sheets. With a knife, straighten sides of chopsticks and line up ½ inch apart. If sticks become too soft to move, return to freezer for several minutes.

5. Bake 8 to 10 minutes, or until firm and very lightly browned. Remove chopsticks to a rack and let cool completely. Brush top third of each chopstick with melted chocolate and refrigerate just until chocolate is firm. Remove from refrigerator as soon as possible because cookie will soften. Store in a tightly covered container in a cool, dry place.

258 CREAM CHEESE RUGELACH

Prep: 25 minutes   Chill: 1 hour   Bake: 13 to 16 minutes   Makes: 64

2 sticks (8 ounces) butter,
  softened
6 ounces cream cheese,
  softened
⅓ cup superfine sugar
3¼ cups cake flour
½ teaspoon salt
½ cup chopped walnuts

⅓ cup finely chopped
  semisweet chocolate or
  mini chocolate chips
½ cup granulated sugar
2 teaspoons cinnamon
½ cup raspberry or blackberry
  preserves

1. In a food processor, combine butter, cream cheese, and superfine sugar. Process until well blended. Add cake flour and salt. Process until dough forms a ball around blades. Wrap in wax paper and refrigerate 1 hour, until firm, or overnight.

2. Preheat oven to 350°F. In a small bowl, combine walnuts, chopped chocolate, granulated sugar, and cinnamon. Mix well.

3. Divide dough into 8 pieces. On a floured work surface, roll out one piece of dough into an 8-inch circle. Spread about 1 tablespoon preserves over dough. Sprinkle about 2 tablespoons walnut-sugar filling on top. Using a pizza wheel or sharp knife, cut into 8 wedges. Beginning at wide end, roll toward point, forming a crescent shape. Repeat with remaining dough, jam, and filling. Place, point sides down, 1 inch apart on greased cookie sheets.

4. Bake 13 to 16 minutes, until golden. Remove to a rack and let cool completely before serving.

---

259 CAT'S TONGUES

Prep: 10 minutes   Bake: 5 to 7 minutes   Makes: about 48

These delicious *langues du chat*, as they are called in French, are wonderfully delicate cookies, a perfect accompaniment to fruit salad, ice cream, or sorbet. The same dough can be baked in rounds and shaped over a rolling pin like lace cookies.

4 tablespoons butter, softened
⅓ cup granulated sugar
1 egg
1 teaspoon vanilla extract

⅔ cup flour
¼ teaspoon grated lemon zest
1 tablespoon powdered sugar

1. Preheat oven to 350°F. In a large bowl, beat butter and granulated sugar with an electric mixer on medium speed until well blended. Beat in egg and vanilla until light and fluffy.

2. Beat in flour and lemon zest until a soft dough forms, scraping down side of bowl frequently with a rubber spatula.

3. For cat's tongues, spoon dough into a pastry bag fitted with a ⅜-inch open tip and pipe 2 inches apart onto greased cookie sheets to form ½ × 3-inch strips. To form rounds, drop by teaspoonfuls 3 inches apart.

4. Bake 5 to 7 minutes, or until golden brown at edges. Let cookies cool 1 minute on sheets, then remove to racks or press over floured rolling pin to curve and let cool completely. When cool, sift powdered sugar over cookies and store in a tightly covered container.

260 DANISH FRIED COOKIES
Prep: 10 minutes   Chill: 30 minutes   Cook: 1 to 2 minutes
Makes: about 50

6 tablespoons butter, softened	¼ teaspoon grated nutmeg
½ cup granulated sugar	¼ teaspoon salt
2 eggs	Vegetable oil, for deep-frying
¼ cup sour cream	Powdered sugar
3 cups cake flour	
½ teaspoon ground cardamom	

1. In a medium bowl, beat butter and sugar with an electric mixer on medium speed until well blended. Beat in eggs, one at a time, and then add sour cream, beating until light and fluffy.

2. Mix flour, cardamom, nutmeg, and salt and beat in gradually on low speed until dough is smooth. Scrape side of bowl frequently with a rubber spatula. Wrap dough and refrigerate at least 30 minutes, until firm.

3. Divide dough into 3 pieces. Between pieces of floured wax paper, roll out one third of dough to make an 8 × 20-inch rectangle. With a sharp knife or pastry wheel, cut rectangle into two 4-inch strips. Cut strips crosswise diagonally at 2-inch intervals. Cut a slit down center of each piece, starting ½ inch from one end and ending ½ inch before other end. Gently lift one end of dough and pull it through slit to twist dough. Twist remaining pieces and set aside. Repeat with remaining dough.

4. In a deep-fat fryer or large heavy saucepan, heat 4 inches of oil to 375°F. on a deep-fat thermometer. Fry dough twists, several at a time, 1 to 2 minutes, or until they are golden brown.

5. With a slotted spatula, remove fried cookies to paper towels to drain. When cookies are cool, sprinkle with powdered sugar and store in a tightly covered container.

261 DANISH ORANGE BARS
Prep: 10 minutes   Bake: 10 to 12 minutes   Makes: about 50

These chocolate-dipped cookies are a holiday favorite. They're also delicious flavored with lemon extract and zest.

1 stick (4 ounces) butter, softened	3 tablespoons grated orange zest
¼ cup sugar	1½ cups flour
1 egg	¼ teaspoon salt
½ teaspoon orange extract	½ cup semisweet chocolate chips, melted

1. Preheat oven to 400°F. In a medium bowl, beat butter and sugar with an electric mixer on medium speed until blended. Beat in egg, orange extract, and orange zest. Mix in flour and salt until a stiff dough forms.

2. On a lightly floured surface, roll dough into an 8 × 5-inch rectangle, about ¼ inch thick. Cut into 2 × 1-inch bars and place 1 inch apart on greased cookie sheets. Reroll scraps if necessary.

3. Bake 10 to 12 minutes, until cookies brown lightly. Let stand 2 minutes, then dip half of each cookie in melted chocolate and place on wax paper on a rack to cool completely.

---

262 GREEK BUTTER BALLS
Prep: 10 minutes   Chill: 1 hour   Bake: 10 to 12 minutes   Makes: about 36

1½ sticks (6 ounces) butter, softened	1 teaspoon vanilla extract
¾ cup superfine sugar	1¾ cups flour
1 egg, at room temperature	1 teaspoon baking powder
3 tablespoons cognac or other brandy	½ cup powdered sugar

1. In a medium bowl, beat butter and superfine sugar with an electric mixer on medium speed until light and fluffy. Beat in egg, cognac, and vanilla.

2. Add flour mixed with baking powder to sugar mixture and beat until blended. Cover and refrigerate dough at least 1 hour, until firm.

3. Preheat oven to 350°F. Shape dough into 1-inch balls and place 1 inch apart on ungreased cookie sheets.

4. Bake 10 to 12 minutes, or until edges just begin to turn golden brown. Remove to a rack to cool slightly, about 10 minutes. Roll in powdered sugar. Let cool completely before serving.

263 ITALIAN FRUIT AND HAZELNUT COOKIES
Prep: 5 minutes   Bake: 15 to 18 minutes   Makes: about 40

Often made with candied rather than dried fruit, these cookies are found in pastry shops and on restaurant cookie samplers throughout Italy. Their Italian name, *brutti ma buoni*, literally means "ugly but good."

1½ cups hazelnuts (about
    6 ounces), coarsely
    chopped
1 cup mixed dried fruit (we
    used sour cherries,
    apricots, and dates)

⅔ cup sugar
3 egg whites
1 teaspoon vanilla extract
¼ teaspoon salt

1. Preheat oven to 350°F. In a food processor, combine hazelnuts, dried fruit, sugar, egg whites, vanilla, and salt. Process, turning machine quickly on and off, until hazelnuts and fruit are finely chopped.

2. Drop by teaspoonfuls 2 inches apart onto generously greased cookie sheets. Bake 15 to 18 minutes, or until golden. Remove cookies immediately to racks and let cool completely. Store in a tightly covered container.

264 JAN HAGELS
Prep: 10 minutes   Bake: 10 to 12 minutes   Makes: 32

⅔ cup sugar
1 stick (4 ounces) butter,
    softened
1 egg
1 teaspoon almond extract

1½ cups flour
¼ teaspoon salt
½ cup sliced natural almonds
½ teaspoon cinnamon

1. Preheat oven to 350°F. Set aside 2 tablespoons sugar. In a medium bowl, beat butter and remaining sugar with an electric mixer on medium speed until well blended. Separate egg; set aside white. Add yolk and almond extract to butter-sugar mixture; beat until light and fluffy.

2. Add flour and salt and beat on low speed until dough is smooth, scraping down side of bowl frequently with a rubber spatula.

3. Flatten dough onto a lightly greased 15½ × 10½-inch jelly-roll pan; top with a sheet of wax paper and roll to fit pan exactly. Remove wax paper. Lightly beat reserved egg white; brush over dough. Sprinkle almonds evenly over dough. Stir together reserved sugar and cinnamon; sprinkle over dough.

4. Bake 10 to 12 minutes, or until golden brown. With a sharp knife, make 3 lengthwise and 7 crosswise cuts through Jan Hagels to divide into 32 rectangles. Let cool completely in pan. Then remove and store in a tightly covered container.

265 LADYFINGERS
Prep: 10 minutes   Bake: 10 to 12 minutes   Makes: about 36

These light, golden cookies are crisper than the packaged variety, but they work just as deliciously in trifles, charlottes, and other recipes where ladyfingers are traditionally used.

2 eggs	1 teaspoon grated lemon zest
¼ teaspoon cream of tartar	½ cup cake flour
⅛ teaspoon salt	Powdered sugar
⅓ cup granulated sugar	

1. Separate eggs. In a medium bowl, combine egg whites and cream of tartar. Set bowl into a pan or larger bowl of hot water for 10 to 15 minutes, or until egg whites reach room temperature.

2. Meanwhile, in a small bowl, combine egg yolks and salt. Beat with an electric mixer on high speed until light. Gradually beat in 3 tablespoons granulated sugar and continue beating until thick and lemon colored. Fold in lemon zest.

3. Preheat oven to 325°F. With clean beaters, beat egg whites and cream of tartar until frothy. Very gradually beat in remaining sugar until soft peaks form when beater is raised.

4. Fold egg yolk mixture and cake flour into beaten whites until batter is just blended. Spoon batter into a pastry bag with a ⅜-inch opening and no decorating tip. Pipe batter onto generously greased cookie sheets to make 4-inch strips, 2 inches apart.

5. Bake 10 to 12 minutes, or until edges just turn golden. Immediately remove ladyfingers to racks and let cool completely. Store in a tightly covered container. Sprinkle with powdered sugar just before serving.

266 KRUMKAKES
Prep: 10 minutes   Bake: 12 to 15 minutes   Makes: about 15

The iron necessary to make these festive cookies is often handed down from generation to generation. If you would like to purchase one and your local housewares store doesn't stock them, see our Mail Order Guide on page 4.

3 eggs	⅔ cup flour
⅓ cup granulated sugar	¼ teaspoon ground cardamom
1 stick (4 ounces) butter, melted	⅛ teaspoon salt
1 teaspoon vanilla extract	¼ cup powdered sugar (optional)
½ teaspoon grated lemon zest	

1. In a large bowl, beat eggs and granulated sugar with an electric mixer on high speed until thick and lemon colored. Set aside 2 tablespoons butter; beat in remaining melted butter, vanilla, and lemon zest.

2. Add flour mixed with cardamom and salt and beat on low speed until dough is smooth, scraping down side of bowl frequently with a rubber spatula.

3. Preheat krumkake iron according to manufacturer's directions. Brush iron with some of reserved melted butter and spoon on about 2½ measuring tablespoons batter. Close and bake krumkake according to manufacturer's directions. Repeat, baking krumkakes until all batter has been used, brushing iron with more butter whenever it seems dry.

4. As they are baked, remove krumkakes to a wire rack to cool. If desired, while still hot, carefully roll into a tube and place, seam side down, on a wire rack until completely cooled. Sprinkle with powdered sugar and store in a tightly covered container.

---

267 ITALIAN FRIED TWISTS
Prep: 10 minutes   Chill: 30 minutes   Fry: 1 to 2 minutes
Makes: 54 twists

These traditional cookies have their roots in a time when ovens were not a part of every home kitchen and cookies were often fried. (Baking was done in shared community ovens.)

3 cups cake flour	2 to 4 tablespoons brandy,
¼ cup granulated sugar	amaretto, or orange-
⅛ teaspoon salt	flavored liqueur
3 tablespoons butter	Vegetable oil for deep-
3 eggs	frying
	Powdered sugar

1. In a medium bowl, combine cake flour, granulated sugar, and salt. With a pastry blender or 2 knives, cut in butter until mixture resembles coarse meal. In a small bowl, beat eggs and 2 tablespoons brandy until well blended. Make a well in center of flour mixture; pour egg mixture into well. With a fork, stir until a smooth dough forms, adding more brandy if necessary. Knead dough into a ball and refrigerate 30 minutes.

2. Divide dough into thirds. Between pieces of floured wax paper, roll out one third of dough to make a 9 × 18-inch rectangle. With a sharp knife or pastry wheel, cut rectangle into 3-inch squares. Cut a lengthwise slit down center of each square starting ½ inch from one corner and ending ½ inch before opposite corner. Gently lift one end of square close to slit and pull it through slit to twist dough. Repeat with remaining squares.

3. In a deep-fat fryer or large heavy saucepan, heat 4 inches of oil to 375°F. on a deep-fat thermometer. Fry dough twists, several at a time, 1 to 2 minutes, or until they are golden brown.

4. With a slotted spatula, remove fried twists to paper towels to drain. When twists are cool, sprinkle with powdered sugar and store in a tightly covered container.

268 CHOCOLATE MADELEINES
Prep: 10 minutes   Bake: 12 to 15 minutes   Makes: 24

1 stick (4 ounces) butter
2 (1-ounce) squares
  unsweetened chocolate,
  chopped
2 eggs
¼ teaspoon cream of tartar

½ cup sugar
½ teaspoon vanilla extract
1 cup flour
¼ teaspoon salt
Sweetened cocoa powder

1. In a small saucepan over very low heat or in a microwave, melt butter and chocolate together, stirring until smooth and blended. Set aside and let cool to room temperature.

2. In a medium bowl, beat eggs with cream of tartar until blended. Set bowl in a pan or larger bowl of hot water for 10 to 15 minutes, or until eggs reach room temperature.

3. Preheat oven to 350°F. Grease and flour madeleine pan. With an electric mixer on medium speed, beat eggs until thick and lemon colored. Gradually beat in sugar and vanilla.

4. With a wire whisk, fold in melted chocolate mixture, flour, and salt until batter is well blended. Spoon 1 tablespoon of batter into each mold of madeleine pans. Cover and refrigerate any remaining batter.

5. Bake 12 to 15 minutes, or until edges are golden brown. Let cookies cool 2 minutes in pans, then remove to racks and let cool completely. Clean and regrease pans; repeat until all batter has been baked. Store madeleines in a tightly covered container. Sprinkle with sweetened cocoa powder just before serving.

269 CURRANT SPICE MADELEINES
Prep: 10 minutes   Bake: 12 to 15 minutes   Makes: 24

These madeleines are a bit less fragile because they have a little baking powder added for leavening.

2 eggs
¼ teaspoon cream of tartar
½ cup firmly packed brown
  sugar
1 teaspoon vanilla extract
1 stick (4 ounces) butter,
  melted and cooled
¾ cup flour

½ teaspoon cinnamon
¼ teaspoon grated nutmeg
¼ teaspoon baking powder
¼ teaspoon salt
⅛ teaspoon ground cloves
¼ cup currants or coarsely
  chopped raisins
Powdered sugar

1. In a medium bowl, beat eggs with cream of tartar until blended. Set bowl in a pan or larger bowl of hot water for 10 to 15 minutes, or until eggs reach room temperature.

2. Preheat oven to 350°F. Grease and flour madeleine pans. With an electric mixer on medium speed, beat eggs until thick and lemon colored. Beat in brown sugar and vanilla.

3. With a wire whisk, fold in melted butter, then flour mixed with cinnamon, nutmeg, baking powder, salt, and cloves until batter is well blended. Fold in currants. Spoon 1 tablespoon of batter into each mold of madeleine pans. Cover and refrigerate any remaining batter.

4. Bake 12 to 15 minutes, or until edges are golden brown. Let cookies cool 2 minutes in pans, then remove to racks and let cool completely. Clean and regrease pans; repeat until all batter has been baked. Store madeleines in a tightly covered container. Sprinkle with powdered sugar just before serving.

---

270 MADELEINES
Prep: 10 minutes   Bake: 12 to 15 minutes   Makes: 18

How could we make French madeleines and not think of Marcel Proust? Almost everyone we know first learned of these sweet little shell-shaped cakes through Proust's description, in *Remembrance of Things Past*, of the "exquisite pleasure that invaded [his] senses" upon sipping a spoonful of tea in which he had dissolved the crumbs of a petite madeleine. This recipe depends entirely upon the air beaten into the eggs for leavening, so be very careful to use clean beaters and bowl and to beat until the egg is very thick and light in color. Madeleines are best eaten freshly baked.

2 eggs	¾ cup flour
¼ teaspoon cream of tartar	1 teaspoon grated lemon zest
½ cup granulated sugar	¼ teaspoon lemon extract
1 stick (4 ounces) butter, melted and cooled	¼ teaspoon salt
	Powdered sugar

1. In a medium bowl, beat eggs with cream of tartar until blended. Set bowl in a pan or larger bowl of hot water for 10 to 15 minutes, or until eggs reach room temperature.

2. Preheat oven to 350°F. Very generously grease and flour 18 molds in madeleine pans. With an electric mixer on high speed, beat eggs until thick and lemon colored. Gradually beat in granulated sugar.

3. With a wire whisk, fold in melted butter, then flour, lemon zest, lemon extract, and salt until batter is well blended. Spoon 1 tablespoon of batter into each mold of madeleine pans. If you don't have enough pans, cover and refrigerate any remaining batter.

4. Bake 12 to 15 minutes, or until edges are golden brown. Let cookies cool 2 minutes in pans, then remove to racks and let cool completely. If necessary, clean and regrease pans; fill with batter and bake as directed above. Repeat until all batter has been baked. Store madeleines in a tightly covered container. Sprinkle with powdered sugar just before serving.

271 MANDELBROT
Prep: 20 minutes   Bake: 18 to 20 minutes   Makes: 60

3½ to 4 cups flour
1¼ cups sugar
2½ teaspoons baking powder
2 teaspoons grated lemon zest
2 teaspoons grated orange zest
Pinch of salt
½ cup vegetable oil

4 eggs
3 tablespoons lemon juice
¼ cup orange juice
1 teaspoon cinnamon
6 tablespoons raspberry or
strawberry jam
⅓ cup chopped almonds

1. Preheat oven to 350°F. In a medium bowl, combine 3½ cups flour, 1 cup sugar, baking powder, lemon zest, orange zest, and salt. Mix with a wooden spoon until blended. Beat in oil, eggs, lemon juice, and orange juice just until dough forms. Add enough remaining flour so dough is not sticky.

2. Stir together remaining ¼ cup sugar with cinnamon until mixed. On a well-floured board, roll one fourth dough into a 12 × 8-inch rectangle. Spread 1½ tablespoons jam over dough, then sprinkle on about 1 tablespoon cinnamon sugar and 1½ tablespoons chopped almonds. Fold in thirds like a business letter. Turn over and place seam side down on greased baking sheet. Repeat 3 times with remaining dough, jam, and almonds.

3. Bake 18 to 20 minutes, until bottom begins to brown. Remove to a rack and let cool before cutting each rectangle crosswise diagonally into fifteen ¾-inch slices.

272 CHOCOLATE LADYFINGERS
Prep: 10 minutes   Bake: 10 to 12 minutes   Makes: about 36

Layer these crisp, chocolatey cookies with sweetened whipped cream for a delicious dessert. Or nibble them out of hand with a cup of hot coffee or cocoa.

2 eggs
¼ teaspoon cream of tartar
⅛ teaspoon salt
½ cup granulated sugar
2 (1-ounce) squares
unsweetened chocolate,
melted

½ teaspoon vanilla extract
½ cup cake flour
Powdered sugar

1. Separate eggs. In a medium bowl, combine egg whites and cream of tartar. Set bowl into a pan or larger bowl of hot water for 10 to 15 minutes, or until egg whites reach room temperature.

2. Meanwhile, in a small bowl, combine yolks and salt. With an electric mixer on high speed, beat egg yolks until light. Gradually beat in ¼ cup granulated sugar and continue beating until thick and lemon colored. Fold in melted chocolate and vanilla.

3. Preheat oven to 325°F. With clean beaters, beat egg whites and cream of tartar until frothy. Very gradually beat in remaining ¼ cup sugar until soft peaks form when beater is raised.

4. Fold chocolate mixture and cake flour into beaten egg whites until batter is just blended. Spoon batter into a pastry bag with a ⅜-inch opening and no decorating tip. Pipe batter onto generously greased cookie sheets to make 4-inch strips, 2 inches apart.

5. Bake 10 to 12 minutes, or until surface looks dry. Immediately remove ladyfingers to racks and let cool completely. Store in a tightly covered container. Sprinkle with powdered sugar just before serving.

---

273 GRANDMA HELEN'S RUGELACH

Prep: 25 minutes   Chill: 1 hour   Bake: 15 to 18 minutes
Makes: about 80

Bonnie's grandmother Helen, who came from Kovno, Russia, was famous for her rugelach. Here's an updated version made quickly in the food processor and lightened with nonfat yogurt.

1 **stick (4 ounces) butter, softened**	1 **tablespoon grated lemon zest**
¼ **cup solid vegetable shortening**	4 **cups flour**
1¾ **cups sugar**	2 **teaspoons baking powder**
3 **eggs**	¾ **cup chopped walnuts**
1 **teaspoon vanilla extract**	½ **cup currants or chopped raisins**
¼ **cup plain nonfat yogurt or sour cream**	1 **tablespoon cinnamon**
1 **tablespoon grated orange zest**	¾ **cup apricot preserves**

1. In a food processor, combine butter, shortening, 1 cup sugar, eggs, vanilla, yogurt, orange zest, and lemon zest. Process until well blended. Add 2 cups flour and baking powder; process until blended. Add 2 cups more flour and process until dough forms a ball around blades. Wrap in wax paper and refrigerate at least 1 hour, until firm, or overnight.

2. Preheat oven to 350°F. In a small bowl, combine walnuts, currants, remaining ¾ cup sugar, and cinnamon. Stir to mix well.

3. Divide dough into 4 equal pieces. On a floured board, roll out one piece into a 20 × 5-inch rectangle. Spread about 3 tablespoons apricot preserves over dough, then sprinkle on about 6 tablespoons walnut-currant mixture. Roll up jelly-roll fashion from a long side. Repeat with remaining dough, preserves, and walnut-currant mixture. Cut each strip diagonally into 1-inch pieces.

4. Place rugelach 1 inch apart on greased cookie sheets. Bake 15 to 18 minutes, until golden. Remove to a rack and let cool completely before serving.

274 MEXICAN ANISE COOKIES
Prep: 10 minutes Bake: 10 to 12 minutes Makes: about 48

These anise-flavored cookies of Mexican origin go particularly well with a cup of espresso or strong coffee.

2 sticks (8 ounces) butter, softened	3¼ cups flour
1½ cups sugar	2 teaspoons baking powder
2 eggs	½ teaspoon salt
½ teaspoon anise extract	2 teaspoons aniseeds, crushed
2 tablespoons brandy	1 teaspoon cinnamon

1. Preheat oven to 350°F. In a medium bowl, beat butter and 1¼ cups sugar with an electric mixer on medium speed until creamy. Beat in eggs, anise extract, and brandy until well blended.

2. Add flour mixed with baking powder, salt, and aniseeds and beat on low speed until well blended. Shape into 1½-inch balls. Place 2 inches apart on ungreased cookie sheets. Using a flat-bottomed glass dipped in flour, flatten each ball slightly into a 2-inch round.

3. In a small bowl, stir together remaining ¼ cup sugar and cinnamon until well mixed. Sprinkle over tops of cookies. Bake 10 to 12 minutes, until light golden. Let cookies cool on sheets 2 minutes, then remove to a rack and let cool completely.

275 MEXICAN WEDDING CAKES
Prep: 10 minutes Chill: 1 hour Bake: 15 to 20 minutes Makes: 48

This is a buttery almond cookie, perfect at any time.

2 sticks (8 ounces) butter, softened	1 teaspoon almond extract
¾ cup plus ½ cup powdered sugar	2 cups flour
1 teaspoon vanilla extract	1 cup finely chopped blanched almonds

1. In a medium bowl, beat butter and ¾ cup powdered sugar with an electric mixer on medium speed until light and fluffy. Beat in vanilla and almond extract.

2. Gradually add flour to sugar mixture and beat until blended. Stir in almonds. Cover and refrigerate dough at least 1 hour, until firm.

3. Preheat oven to 325°F. Shape dough into 1-inch balls and place 1 inch apart on ungreased cookie sheets. Bake 15 to 20 minutes, or until edges just begin to turn golden brown.

4. Remove cookies to a rack to cool slightly, about 10 minutes. Roll in remaining ½ cup powdered sugar. Let cool completely before serving.

276 MEXICAN CINNAMON CRISPS
Prep: 10 minutes   Fry: 1 to 2 minutes   Makes: 48

8 (6-inch) flour tortillas	Vegetable oil, for deep-
¼ cup sugar	frying
1 tablespoon cinnamon	

1. Cut tortillas into 6 wedges each. In a small bowl, stir together sugar and cinnamon until well mixed.

2. In a large heavy saucepan or deep-fat fryer, heat 4 inches oil to 375°F. on a deep-fat thermometer. Fry tortilla triangles, several at a time, 1 to 2 minutes, or until golden brown.

3. With a slotted spatula, remove fried triangles to paper towels to drain. Immediately sprinkle with cinnamon sugar. Let cool completely; store in a tightly covered container.

---

277 CINNAMONY MEXICAN BUTTER COOKIES
Prep: 10 minutes   Bake: 20 to 25 minutes   Makes: about 36

2 sticks (8 ounces) butter, softened	2 cups flour
½ cup powdered sugar	2 teaspoons baking powder
1 teaspoon vanilla extract	2 teaspoons cinnamon
	½ cup granulated sugar

1. Preheat oven to 350°F. In a medium bowl, beat butter and powdered sugar with an electric mixer on medium speed until creamy. Beat in vanilla.

2. Add flour mixed with baking powder and 1½ teaspoons cinnamon and beat until well blended. Shape dough into 1-inch balls. Place 2 inches apart on ungreased cookie sheets. Using bottom of a glass, flatten each ball into a 2-inch circle.

3. Bake 20 to 25 minutes, until cookies are lightly browned. Let stand 2 minutes.

4. In a small bowl, stir together granulated sugar and ½ teaspoon cinnamon. Dip each cookie into cinnamon sugar, then transfer to a rack and let cool completely.

278 PIZZELLES
Prep: 10 minutes   Bake: 12 to 15 minutes   Makes: about 16

A monogrammed pizzelle iron is a traditional Italian wedding gift.

3 eggs
½ cup granulated sugar
1 stick (4 ounces) butter, melted
1 tablespoon vanilla extract

1⅔ cups flour
1½ teaspoons baking powder
⅛ teaspoon salt
¼ cup powdered sugar (optional)

1. In a large bowl, beat eggs and granulated sugar with an electric mixer on high speed until thick and lemon colored. Set aside 2 tablespoons butter; beat in remaining melted butter and vanilla.

2. Add flour mixed with baking powder and salt and beat on low speed until dough is smooth, scraping down side of bowl frequently with a rubber spatula.

3. Preheat and grease pizzelle iron according to manufacturer's directions. Brush iron with some of reserved melted butter; spoon about 1 heaping tablespoon batter in center of iron. Close and bake pizzelle according to manufacturer's directions. Repeat, baking pizzelles until all batter has been used, brushing iron with more butter whenever it seems dry.

4. As they are baked, remove pizzelles to a wire rack to cool completely. Sprinkle with powdered sugar if desired and store in a tightly covered container.

279 SCOTCH SHORTBREAD
Prep: 5 minutes   Bake: 20 to 25 minutes   Makes: 24

Traditional shortbread is made without the use of a mixer.

2 sticks (8 ounces) butter, softened
½ cup plus 2 tablespoons sugar

½ teaspoon vanilla extract
2 cups flour
¼ teaspoon salt

1. Preheat oven to 325°F. In a medium bowl with a wooden spoon, mix butter and ½ cup sugar together until light and fluffy. Beat in vanilla. Stir in flour and salt.

2. Divide dough in half. Press each half evenly over bottom of a 9-inch pie pan. Crimp edges and prick all over with a fork. Using a knife, cut each into 12 wedges. Sprinkle 1 tablespoon sugar evenly over each shortbread.

3. Bake 20 to 25 minutes, until pale golden but not brown. Let cool in pan on a wire rack 5 minutes, then recut into wedges. Transfer to rack and let cool completely.

280 RASPBERRY RIBBONS
Prep: 10 minutes   Bake: 15 to 20 minutes   Makes: 48

These jam-filled cookies originated in Denmark. They're a colorful addition to any holiday tray.

2 sticks (8 ounces) butter, softened	2¼ cups flour
½ cup granulated sugar	¼ teaspoon salt
1 egg	½ cup raspberry jam
2 teaspoons vanilla extract	⅔ cup powdered sugar
	2 tablespoons half-and-half

1. Preheat oven to 375°F. In a medium bowl, beat butter, granulated sugar, egg, and 1 teaspoon vanilla with an electric mixer on medium speed until well blended.

2. Add flour and salt and beat until a smooth dough forms. On a lightly floured surface, shape one fourth of dough into a 12 × 1-inch strip about ¼ inch thick. Repeat with remaining dough. Place on an ungreased cookie sheet. Using your finger or a chopstick, make an indentation down the central length of each strip.

3. Bake 10 minutes. Gently spoon raspberry jam into groove and return to oven 5 to 10 minutes, until edges brown lightly. Remove to a rack and let cool for 2 minutes.

4. In a small bowl, stir together powdered sugar, half-and-half, and remaining 1 teaspoon vanilla. Drizzle glaze over hot cookies. Let cool, then cut strips diagonally into 1-inch slices.

281 SCANDINAVIAN BUTTER COOKIES
Prep: 20 minutes   Bake: 10 to 12 minutes   Makes: 24

These traditional cookies get most of their sweetness from their crisp sugar coating.

1 stick (4 ounces) butter, softened	2 tablespoons ice water
1¾ cups flour	1 teaspoon almond extract
½ cup sugar	¼ teaspoon salt

1. Preheat oven to 350°F. In a medium bowl, beat butter, flour, 2 tablespoons sugar, ice water, almond extract, and salt with an electric mixer on medium speed just until well blended.

2. Divide dough into 24 pieces. Spread remaining sugar on a piece of wax paper. With palms of hands, roll each piece of dough to make a 7-inch rope. Roll ropes in sugar and shape into figure eights. Set 2 inches apart on lightly greased cookie sheets.

3. Bake 10 to 12 minutes, or until golden brown. Let cookies cool 2 minutes on sheets, then remove to racks and let cool completely. Store in a tightly covered container.

282 ROSETTES
Prep: 10 minutes   Cook: 10 to 15 minutes total   Makes: 18

Although these crisp golden cookies are often associated with the holidays, they make a festive appearance at any occasion, and once you have the equipment they are not hard to make. They are best if eaten the same day they are made.

¼ cup flour
¼ cup cornstarch
1 tablespoon granulated sugar
½ teaspoon cinnamon
⅛ teaspoon salt
1 egg

¼ cup milk
2 tablespoons butter, melted
1 teaspoon vanilla extract
  Vegetable oil for deep-
    frying
¼ cup powdered sugar

1. In a medium bowl, combine flour, cornstarch, granulated sugar, cinnamon, and salt. Stir to mix well. Blend in egg, milk, melted butter, and vanilla until a smooth batter forms.

2. In a large heavy saucepan or deep-fat fryer, heat 4 inches oil to 375°F. on a deep-frying thermometer. Preheat rosette iron in oil according to manufacturer's directions.

3. Dip hot rosette iron into batter, being careful not to go over top of iron. Then dip it into hot oil until rosette is golden, about 30 to 45 seconds. Gently remove rosette from iron with a fork and place on paper towels to drain. Repeat until all batter has been used. When rosettes are cool, sprinkle with powdered sugar.

283 RUSSIAN RYE COOKIES
Prep: 10 minutes   Chill: 3 hours   Bake: 12 to 15 minutes
Makes: about 36

½ cup sugar
1½ sticks (6 ounces) butter,
    softened
¼ cup dark corn syrup
1 egg
1 teaspoon vanilla extract
1 cup all-purpose flour
1 cup rye flour

½ teaspoon baking powder
1 teaspoon cinnamon
¼ teaspoon grated nutmeg
¼ teaspoon freshly ground
    black pepper
⅛ teaspoon salt
  Whole blanched almonds
    (optional)

1. Set aside 1 tablespoon of sugar. In a medium bowl, beat remaining sugar and butter with an electric mixer on medium speed until well blended. Beat in corn syrup, egg, and vanilla until light and fluffy.

2. Mix all-purpose flour, rye flour, baking powder, cinnamon, nutmeg, pepper, and salt. Add to butter mixture and beat on low speed until dough is smooth, scraping down side of bowl frequently with a rubber spatula. Wrap and refrigerate dough 3 hours, until firm.

3. Preheat oven to 350°F. Between pieces of wax paper, roll out dough ¼ inch thick. Cut with 2½-inch fluted round or square cookie cutters. Reroll scraps to make additional cookies. Place cookies 2 inches apart on lightly greased cookie sheets. Place an almond in center of each, if desired. Sprinkle reserved sugar over tops of cookies.

4. Bake 12 to 15 minutes, or until edges are golden brown. Let cookies cool 2 minutes on sheets, then remove to racks and let cool completely. Store in a tightly covered container.

---

284 SCHNECKEN
Prep: 20 minutes   Bake: 8 to 10 minutes   Makes: 36

Schnecken means snails, referring to the coiled shape of these cookies. It is more fun if you have help to roll these little cinnamon snails, the younger the better.

1½ sticks (6 ounces) butter, softened	2¼ cups flour
½ cup firmly packed brown sugar	¼ teaspoon salt
1 egg	2 tablespoons granulated sugar
½ teaspoon vanilla extract	½ teaspoon cinnamon
	72 whole cloves (optional)

1. Preheat oven to 350°F. In a large bowl, beat butter and brown sugar with an electric mixer on medium speed until light and fluffy. Add egg and vanilla and beat until blended. Beat in flour and salt until dough is smooth, scraping down side of bowl frequently with a rubber spatula.

2. Divide dough in half. Set aside half of dough, covered with plastic wrap. From remaining dough, pinch off 18 slightly rounded measuring tablespoonfuls of dough and roll with your hands into 8-inch ropes.

3. In a pie plate or on a piece of wax paper, stir together granulated sugar and cinnamon until mixed. Brush dough ropes lightly with water and roll in cinnamon sugar mixture. Roll up in a spiral and place 2 inches apart on lightly greased cookie sheets. Repeat with remaining dough. If desired, place 2 cloves, points up, at outside end of snail to resemble antennae.

4. Bake schnecken 8 to 10 minutes, or until golden brown. Let cookies cool 2 minutes on sheets, then remove to racks and let cool completely. Store in a tightly covered container.

285 SWISS HONEY ALMOND COOKIES

Prep: 20 minutes   Chill: 3 hours   Bake: 20 minutes   Makes: 48

A holiday tradition in Switzerland, where they are called *biberli*, these cookies are very hard when first baked but mellow and soften after several days' storage.

½ cup honey	½ teaspoon ground ginger
¼ cup firmly packed brown sugar	¼ teaspoon ground anise
	¼ teaspoon ground coriander
1 egg	¼ teaspoon salt
2 tablespoons brandy	⅛ teaspoon ground cloves
1 teaspoon grated lemon zest	Honey Almond Filling
2 cups flour	(recipe follows)
½ teaspoon baking soda	½ cup powdered sugar
1 teaspoon cinnamon	4 teaspoons lemon juice

1. In a medium bowl, beat honey, brown sugar, egg, brandy, and lemon zest with an electric mixer on medium speed until well blended. Mix together flour, baking soda, cinnamon, ginger, anise, coriander, salt, and cloves. Add to honey mixture and beat on low speed until dough is smooth, scraping down side of bowl frequently with a rubber spatula. Divide dough in half; wrap and refrigerate at least 3 hours, or until firm. (Meanwhile, prepare filling.)

2. Preheat oven to 350°F. Between pieces of generously floured wax paper, roll out each piece of dough to make a 10 × 6-inch rectangle. Cut dough rectangles in half lengthwise to make two 10 × 3-inch strips from each large rectangle.

3. Place one fourth of filling lengthwise in a mound down center of each strip. Moisten lengthwise edges of pastry. Lift pastry edges of one strip to cover filling and overlap slightly; roll over, seam side down. Repeat with remaining strips to make 4 rolls. Cut each roll crosswise into 12 cookies. Place cookies, seam side down, 2 inches apart on well-greased baking sheets.

4. Bake 20 minutes, or until edges begin to brown. Remove cookies to racks immediately.

5. Meanwhile, stir together powdered sugar and lemon juice to make a glaze. Brush glaze over hot cookies as soon as they have been removed to racks. Let cool completely. Store in a tightly covered container. Cookies are best if allowed to ripen 3 or 4 days before serving.

HONEY ALMOND FILLING
Makes about 2 cups

1½ cups blanched almonds
½ cup sugar
¼ cup packed dried apricots
¼ cup honey

2 teaspoons grated lemon zest
2 tablespoons brandy
1 teaspoon almond extract

In a food processor, combine almonds, sugar, dried apricots, honey, lemon zest, brandy, and almond extract. Process until almonds and apricots are finely chopped.

---

286 SUGAR ZWIEBACK
Prep: 10 minutes   Rise: 1 hour   Bake: 40 to 42 minutes
Stand: 45 minutes   Makes: 48

These zwieback have a crisp sugary crust and are delicately spiced with nutmeg.

1 cup milk
4 tablespoons butter, cut into chunks
½ teaspoon salt
⅔ cup sugar
1 (¼-ounce) envelope active dry yeast

¼ cup lukewarm water (105° to 115°)
1 egg
4 to 4½ cups flour
½ teaspoon grated nutmeg

1. Heat milk in a small saucepan just until bubbles form around edge of pan. Remove from heat; stir in butter and salt. Set aside 2 teaspoons sugar. Stir remaining sugar into milk mixture. Let cool to room temperature.

2. In a large bowl, combine yeast and warm water. Set aside 5 minutes for yeast to soften. Beat cooled milk mixture, egg, 4 cups flour, and nutmeg into yeast mixture with a wooden spoon or dough hook of an electric mixer.

3. Knead dough in bowl, adding more flour if necessary, until a smooth, soft dough forms. Divide dough into 8 balls 3 inches in diameter. Place balls 4 inches apart on lightly greased cookie sheets; pat into 4-inch rounds. Brush tops of rounds with water and sprinkle with reserved sugar. Set aside, lightly covered with kitchen towels, about 1 hour, or until doubled in size.

4. Preheat oven to 350°F. Bake raised rounds 30 minutes, or until golden brown. Remove from oven; leave oven on. Let cool on sheets 10 to 15 minutes, or until cool enough to handle.

5. With a serrated knife, cut each round into six ½-inch slices. Place slices, cut sides down, on cookie sheets and return to oven 5 minutes. Turn slices and bake 5 to 7 minutes longer, or until golden on both sides. Turn off heat and leave zwieback in unopened oven until cool, about 45 minutes. Remove zwieback to racks and let cool completely. Store in a tightly covered container.

287   PLAIN ZWIEBACK
Prep: 10 minutes   Rise: 1 hour   Bake: 40 to 42 minutes
Stand: 45 minutes   Makes: 48

Zwieback means "twice baked." Thrifty German cooks sliced leftover breakfast rolls and toasted them for snacks and to serve with afternoon tea.

1 cup milk	1 (¼-ounce) envelope active
2 tablespoons butter, cut into	dry yeast
chunks	¼ cup lukewarm water (105° to
¼ cup honey	115°)
½ teaspoon salt	4 to 4½ cups flour

1. Heat milk in a small saucepan just until bubbles form around edge of pan. Remove from heat; stir in butter, honey, and salt. Set aside and let cool to room temperature.

2. In a large bowl, combine yeast and lukewarm water. Set aside 5 minutes for yeast to soften. Add cooled milk mixture to softened yeast and beat in 4 cups flour with a wooden spoon or dough hook of an electric mixer.

3. Knead dough in bowl, adding up to ½ cup more flour if necessary, until a smooth, soft dough forms. Divide dough into 8 balls 3 inches in diameter. Place balls 4 inches apart on lightly greased cookie sheets; pat into 4-inch rounds. Set aside, lightly covered with kitchen towels, about 1 hour, or until doubled in size.

4. Preheat oven to 350°F. Bake raised rounds 30 minutes, or until golden brown. Remove from oven; leave oven on. Let cool on sheets 10 to 15 minutes, or until cool enough to handle.

5. With a serrated knife, cut each round into six ½-inch slices. Place slices, cut sides down, on cookie sheets and return to oven 5 minutes. Turn slices and bake 5 to 7 minutes longer, or until golden on both sides. Turn off heat and leave zwieback in unopened oven until cool, about 45 minutes. Store in a tightly covered container.

---

288   SPANISH ANISE BISCUITS
Prep: 10 minutes   Chill: 30 minutes   Bake: 8 to 10 minutes
Makes: about 32

These anise-scented cookies are sometimes called olive oil biscuits.

½ cup sugar	1 egg
1½ cups flour	¼ cup light olive oil or other
½ teaspoon aniseed	vegetable oil
⅛ teaspoon salt	2 tablespoons ice water

1. Reserve 2 tablespoons of sugar. In a medium bowl, stir together remaining sugar, flour, aniseed, and salt; make a well in center. In a cup, combine egg, oil, and ice water; pour into well in flour mixture. With a fork, stir until a smooth dough forms. Knead dough into a ball and refrigerate 30 minutes.

2. Preheat oven to 400°F. Between pieces of wax paper, roll out dough ¼ inch thick. Cut out with a 2-inch round cutter. Reroll scraps to make additional cookies.

3. Place cookies 2 inches apart on lightly greased cookie sheets. Sprinkle reserved sugar on top. Bake 8 to 10 minutes, or until edges are golden brown. Let cookies cool 2 minutes on sheets, then remove to racks and let cool completely. Store in a tightly covered container.

---

289 SPECULAAS
Prep: 20 minutes   Chill: 2 hours   Bake: 10 to 15 minutes
Makes: about 28

These almond-flavored cookies hail from Holland, where they are usually shaped in large wooden molds.

1 **stick (4 ounces) butter, softened**	¼ **teaspoon ground mace or grated nutmeg**
¾ **cup sugar**	⅛ **teaspoon salt**
1½ **teaspoons vanilla extract**	½ **cup sliced blanched almonds**
½ **teaspoon almond extract**	**Whole blanched almonds**
1½ **cups flour**	**(optional)**
1½ **teaspoons baking powder**	

1. In a medium bowl, beat butter and sugar with an electric mixer on medium speed until well blended. Beat in vanilla and almond extract until light and fluffy.

2. Add flour mixed with baking powder, mace, and salt and beat on low speed until dough is smooth, scraping down side of bowl frequently with a rubber spatula. Wrap and refrigerate dough 2 to 3 hours, until firm.

3. Preheat oven to 350°F. For molded cookies, break off pieces of dough and press into well-floured speculaas molds; unmold 2 inches apart onto lightly greased cookie sheets. Or roll out dough ¼ inch thick between pieces of wax paper. Cut with 3-inch round cookie cutters or cut into 3-inch squares and place 2 inches apart on lightly greased cookie sheets. Reroll scraps to make additional cookies. If desired, decorate with whole almonds.

4. Bake 12 to 15 minutes for molded cookies; 10 to 12 minutes for rolled ones. Let cookies cool 2 minutes on sheets, then remove to racks and let cool completely. Store in a tightly covered container.

290 TUILES

Prep: 5 minutes   Bake: 6 to 8 minutes   Makes: about 24

These crisp almond cookies mix up in a snap. The trick is to bake no more than six at a time, because they must be formed quickly into their traditional *tuile*, or tile, shape while they are still soft, as soon as they are removed from the oven.

2 egg whites	**¼** teaspoon vanilla extract
½ cup superfine sugar	**4** tablespoons butter, melted
⅛ teaspoon salt	**¼** cup cake flour
¼ teaspoon almond extract	**¾** cup chopped almonds

1. Preheat oven to 400°F. Grease and lightly flour 2 cookie sheets. In a medium bowl, combine egg whites, sugar, salt, almond extract, and vanilla. Beat with an electric mixer on low speed until foamy.

2. Slowly add melted butter, mixing until well blended. Gently stir in cake flour until smooth. Stir in almonds. Batter will be thin.

3. Drop 2 teaspoonfuls batter at least 3 inches apart onto prepared cookie sheets and spread into 3-inch circles with back of a spoon. Make only 4 at a time, to allow enough time to shape them. Bake 6 to 8 minutes, or until golden. Remove from baking sheet and immediately drape over a rolling pin or roll of aluminum foil, pressing down for a few moments, until cookie curves and hardens. (If cookie hardens before shaping, return to oven for 1 minute to soften.) Repeat with remaining batter. When cool, store in airtight container.

Chapter 12

Holiday and Celebration Cookies

Cookies have been associated with holidays for centuries. Sometimes a special cookie was the only thing that differentiated a holiday meal from the usual peasant fare. These traditional cookies were the most likely recipes to make the journey to the New World and the first to be produced here as soon as the ingredients could be found. As children, we noticed that one of the first signs of an approaching holiday was a sweet, spicy aroma and increased activity in the kitchen. A stack of special tins would appear from their rest-of-the-year hiding place, and mounds of special treats would be carefully packed between layers of wax paper for their once-a-year appearance at Christmas and other holiday celebrations.

In addition to ethnic cookie traditions, most families have developed a list of cookies that are their own special celebrations. It just wouldn't be a holiday if those cookies didn't appear on the table, and everyone would be very surprised if they were baked at any other time of the year.

Celebration cookies don't have to fit into any of the current requirements for inclusion in a family's menus. They don't have to be fast and easy to make; they don't have to be low in fat or sodium; and most of all, they don't have to be low in sugar or calories. Celebration cookies are special. They are symbolic—food for the soul as well as the body. Without an occasional cookie-filled celebration, life would be very dull indeed. We hope we have included your favorite celebration cookies in this chapter and that you will want to add some of ours to your list of family traditions.

291   CANDY CANES
Prep: 20 minutes   Bake: 8 to 10 minutes   Makes: 30

It is important to work quickly when rolling and twisting the doughs for these cookie candy canes. If the rolls are allowed to dry out before twisting, they will break.

1½ sticks (6 ounces) butter, softened	¼ teaspoon salt
¾ cup sugar	1 (1-ounce) square unsweetened chocolate, melted
1 egg	
2 teaspoons vanilla extract	2 tablespoons powdered sugar
2¼ cups flour	

1. Preheat oven to 350°F. In a large bowl, beat butter and sugar with an electric mixer on medium speed until light and fluffy. Add egg and vanilla and beat until smooth. Beat in flour and salt until dough is smooth, scraping down side of bowl frequently with a rubber spatula.

2. Divide dough in half. Stir melted chocolate and powdered sugar into one half until color is even. Divide doughs in half again. Set aside half of each color dough, covered with plastic wrap. From remaining doughs make fifteen 6-inch ropes of each color, using about 1 heaping measuring teaspoon dough for each.

3. Place pairs of dough ropes side by side, using one light and one dark for each. Twist ropes together and place 2 inches apart on lightly greased cookie sheets, curving one end to resemble a candy cane. Repeat with remaining dough.

4. Bake candy canes 8 to 10 minutes, or until golden brown. Let cookies cool 2 minutes on sheets, then remove to racks and let cool completely. Store in a tightly covered container.

---

292   CRISPY ANISE COOKIES
Prep: 10 minutes   Bake: 12 to 14 minutes   Makes: about 24

2 eggs	½ teaspoon baking powder
¾ cup superfine sugar	¼ teaspoon salt
¼ teaspoon anise extract	1 teaspoon aniseeds, crushed
1½ cups flour	

1. Preheat oven to 350°F. In a medium bowl, beat eggs with an electric mixer on medium speed until foamy. Gradually add superfine sugar and anise extract and continue beating until thick and lemon colored.

2. In another medium bowl, stir together flour, baking powder, salt, and aniseeds until mixed. Gently fold spiced flour into sugar mixture until blended. Drop by tablespoonfuls 2 inches apart onto greased cookie sheets.

3. Bake 12 to 14 minutes, until cookies are light golden. Remove to a rack and let cool completely.

293 CHOCOLATE LEAF COOKIES

Prep: 20 minutes   Bake: 6 to 8 minutes   Makes: about 48

Beautiful to look at and delicious to eat, these chocolate-coated leaf cookies will be a hit any time. Use a leaf stencil, available at cookware shops, or make one out of heavy cardboard.

2 sticks (8 ounces) butter, softened
⅓ cup superfine sugar
1 teaspoon almond extract
½ teaspoon vanilla extract

1½ cups finely ground blanched almonds
1 cup flour
6 (1-ounce) squares semisweet chocolate, chopped

1. Preheat oven to 375°F. In a medium bowl, beat butter and superfine sugar with an electric mixer on medium speed until light and fluffy. Beat in almond extract and vanilla. Add ground almonds and flour and beat until blended.

2. Place a 4½-inch leaf stencil on an ungreased cookie sheet. With a metal spatula or knife, spread 1 level tablespoon dough over stencil. Remove excess dough, then gently lift stencil, leaving cookie on sheet. Repeat with remaining dough, leaving 1½ inches between leaves.

3. Bake 6 to 8 minutes, until edges are just golden. Let stand 2 minutes on sheet, then remove to a rack and let cool completely.

4. Melt chocolate in top of a double boiler over hot water or in a microwave. Spread melted chocolate over bottoms of leaves. Let chocolate cool and set before storing cookies in an airtight tin between layers of wax paper.

294 RICH ANISE COOKIES

Prep: 10 minutes   Bake: 12 to 15 minutes   Makes: about 36

These licorice-flavored cookies practically melt in your mouth.

1 stick (4 ounces) plus 2 tablespoons butter, softened
⅔ cup sugar
2 eggs

½ teaspoon anise extract
2 cups flour
2 teaspoons baking powder
½ teaspoon salt
1 teaspoon aniseeds, crushed

1. Preheat oven to 350°F. In a medium bowl, beat butter and sugar with an electric mixer on medium speed until creamy. Beat in eggs and anise extract until mixed.

2. Add flour mixed with baking powder, salt, and aniseeds and beat on low speed until well blended. Using 2 teaspoonfuls of dough per cookie, shape into 2-inch-long ovals. Place 1 inch apart on ungreased cookie sheets.

3. Bake 12 to 15 minutes, until cookies are lightly browned. Let cool on sheets 2 minutes, then remove to a rack and let cool completely.

295 CHOCOLATE NUT MERINGUES
Prep: 10 minutes   Bake: 50 minutes   Makes: about 42

Both kids and adults will love these chocolate-and-nut-studded cookies. Since they contain no flour, they are particularly appropriate for Passover.

Vegetable cooking spray	¾ cup semisweet chocolate
2 egg whites	chips, finely chopped
⅛ teaspoon cream of tartar	½ cup finely chopped nuts:
½ cup superfine sugar	almonds, walnuts, and/or
1 teaspoon vanilla extract	pecans

1. Preheat oven to 275°F. Line 2 cookie sheets with foil and lightly coat foil with vegetable cooking spray.

2. In a medium bowl, beat egg whites and cream of tartar with an electric mixer on medium speed until soft peaks form. Turn mixer to high and gradually beat in sugar until glossy, stiff peaks form. Beat in vanilla. Gently but quickly fold in chocolate and nuts. Drop by teaspoonfuls 1 inch apart onto prepared cookie sheets.

3. Bake 25 minutes. Reduce heat to 250°F. and bake 25 minutes longer. Remove to a rack and let cool completely before storing in an airtight tin.

296 CRANBERRY ORANGE BUTTER COOKIES
Prep: 10 minutes   Chill: 1 hour   Bake: 8 to 10 minutes
Makes: about 48

2 sticks (8 ounces) butter, softened	2½ cups flour
	1 teaspoon baking powder
¾ cup firmly packed dark brown sugar	¼ teaspoon salt
	¾ cup dried cranberries, finely chopped (about 3 ounces)
1 egg	
1 teaspoon vanilla extract	¾ cup finely chopped walnuts
½ teaspoon orange extract	½ cup powdered sugar

1. In a medium bowl, beat butter and brown sugar with an electric mixer on medium speed until light and fluffy. Beat in egg, vanilla, and orange extract.

2. Add flour mixed with baking powder and salt and beat on low speed until blended. Mix in dried cranberries and walnuts. Cover and refrigerate at least 1 hour, until firm.

3. Preheat oven to 375°F. Shape dough into 1-inch balls and place 1 inch apart on ungreased cookie sheets. Bake 8 to 10 minutes, or until edges just begin to turn golden brown. Let stand 2 minutes, then roll in powdered sugar, transfer to a rack, and let cool completely.

297 CRANBERRY ORANGE MERINGUES
Prep: 10 minutes   Bake: 50 minutes   Makes: about 42

Because they contain no flour or added fat, meringues provide a treat lower in calories than traditional dessert fare. We like to serve these delicious cranberry-orange morsels at Thanksgiving after pie and coffee.

Vegetable cooking spray
2 egg whites
⅛ teaspoon cream of tartar
⅔ cup superfine sugar
½ teaspoon vanilla extract
½ teaspoon orange extract

¾ cup dried cranberries, finely chopped (about 3 ounces)
½ cup finely chopped pecans
1 tablespoon grated orange zest

1. Preheat oven to 275°F. Line 2 cookie sheets with foil and lightly coat foil with vegetable cooking spray.

2. In a medium bowl, beat egg whites and cream of tartar with an electric mixer on medium speed until soft peaks form. Turn mixer to high and gradually beat in superfine sugar until glossy, stiff peaks form. Beat in vanilla and orange extract. Gently but quickly fold in cranberries, pecans, and orange zest. Drop by teaspoonfuls 1 inch apart onto prepared cookie sheets.

3. Bake 25 minutes. Reduce oven temperature to 250°F. and bake 25 minutes longer. Remove meringues to a rack and let cool completely. Store in an airtight tin.

298 DATE-NUT MERINGUES
Prep: 10 minutes   Bake: 50 minutes   Makes: about 42

Vegetable cooking spray
2 egg whites
⅛ teaspoon cream of tartar
⅔ cup superfine sugar

1 teaspoon vanilla extract
½ cup finely chopped pitted dates
⅓ cup finely chopped walnuts

1. Preheat oven to 275°F. Line 2 cookie sheets with foil and coat foil with vegetable cooking spray.

2. In a medium bowl, beat egg whites and cream of tartar with an electric mixer on medium speed until soft peaks form. Turn mixer to high and gradually beat in superfine sugar until glossy, stiff peaks form. Beat in vanilla. Gently but quickly fold in dates and walnuts. Drop by teaspoonfuls 1 inch apart onto prepared cookie sheets.

3. Bake 25 minutes. Reduce heat to 250°F. and bake 25 minutes longer. Remove to a rack and let cool completely. Store in an airtight tin.

299 FABULOUS FRUITCAKE COOKIES

Prep: 15 minutes   Bake: 25 to 30 minutes   Makes: about 36

Dried blueberries and cherries along with an assortment of spices and a generous dose of brandy help make these cookies exceptionally flavorful.

4 tablespoons butter, softened	¼ cup brandy or rum
½ cup firmly packed dark brown sugar	2 tablespoons nonfat plain yogurt
2 tablespoons unsulphured molasses	1¾ cups flour
½ teaspoon cinnamon	1½ teaspoons baking soda
½ teaspoon ground ginger	¼ teaspoon salt
½ teaspoon ground allspice	1¼ cups dried blueberries or currants
¼ teaspoon grated nutmeg	1¼ cups dried cherries
¼ teaspoon ground mace	½ cup raisins
2 eggs	2 cups chopped almonds

1. Preheat oven to 275°F. In a medium bowl, beat butter and brown sugar with an electric mixer on medium speed until light and fluffy. Beat in molasses, cinnamon, ginger, allspice, nutmeg, and mace until blended. Add eggs, brandy, and yogurt and blend well.

2. Add 1½ cups of flour, baking soda, and salt and beat until blended. In a medium bowl, toss blueberries, cherries, raisins, and almonds with remaining ¼ cup flour; stir into dough until well mixed.

3. Drop by teaspoonfuls 2 inches apart onto greased cookie sheets. Bake 25 to 30 minutes, until set. Remove to a rack and let cool completely.

---

300 GREEK HOLIDAY COOKIES

Prep: 20 minutes   Bake: 15 to 20 minutes   Makes: 36

4 tablespoons butter, softened	2 cups cake flour
¾ cup powdered sugar	2 teaspoons baking powder
1 egg	¼ teaspoon salt
2 tablespoons half-and-half or milk	1 egg yolk, lightly beaten
	⅓ cup sesame seeds

1. Preheat oven to 375°F. In a medium bowl, beat butter and powdered sugar with an electric mixer on medium speed until light and fluffy. Beat in egg and half-and-half.

2. Add cake flour mixed with baking powder and salt and beat on low speed until blended. Divide one fourth of dough into 9 portions. On a lightly floured surface, roll each portion into a thin rope about 6 inches long, fold in half, and twist like a corkscrew. If dough is sticky, add a bit more flour.

3. Brush with egg yolk and sprinkle sesame seeds on top. Place 2 inches apart on ungreased cookie sheets. Bake 15 to 20 minutes, or until golden. Remove to a rack and let cool completely.

301 GINGERBREAD MEN AND WOMEN

Prep: 15 minutes   Stand: 30 minutes   Chill: 15 minutes
Bake: 10 to 12 minutes   Makes: about 36

This versatile dough is good for all sorts of holiday decorations as well as the traditional gingerbread men and women. We used large cutters to make cookies that were about 4 × 6 inches.

¾ cup solid vegetable shortening, melted	1 tablespoon ground ginger
¾ cup sugar	1 teaspoon cinnamon
¾ cup light molasses	¼ teaspoon salt
3 cups flour	Currants (optional)

1. In a large bowl, beat shortening, sugar, and molasses with an electric mixer on medium speed until well blended. Beat in flour mixed with ginger, cinnamon, and salt until dough is smooth, scraping down side of bowl frequently with a rubber spatula. Cover dough and set aside at room temperature 30 minutes.

2. Preheat oven to 350°F. Between pieces of wax paper, roll out dough ¼ inch thick. Place in freezer 15 minutes for easier handling. Cut out 6-inch gingerbread men and women with cookie cutters.

3. Place cookies 2 inches apart on lightly greased cookie sheets. Decorate with currants, if desired. Reroll scraps to make additional cookies. Place dough in freezer for a few minutes whenever it becomes too soft to handle.

4. Bake 10 to 12 minutes, or until edges start to brown. Let cookies cool 2 minutes on sheets, then remove to racks and let cool completely. Store in a tightly covered container.

---

302 ORANGE PECAN HOLIDAY KISSES

Prep: 10 minutes   Bake: 20 to 25 minutes   Makes: about 48

1½ sticks (6 ounces) butter, softened	½ teaspoon orange extract
1 (3-ounce) package cream cheese, softened	2 teaspoons grated orange zest
	2 cups cake flour
¾ cup granulated sugar	¼ teaspoon salt
½ teaspoon vanilla extract	½ cup finely chopped pecans
	½ cup powdered sugar

1. Preheat oven to 300°F. In a medium bowl, beat butter, cream cheese, and granulated sugar with an electric mixer on medium speed until light and fluffy. Beat in vanilla, orange extract, and orange zest.

2. Add cake flour and salt and beat on low speed until blended. Stir in pecans. Drop by teaspoonfuls 2 inches apart onto ungreased cookie sheets. Bake 20 to 25 minutes, until set but not browned. Let stand 2 minutes on cookie sheets, then roll in powdered sugar. Transfer to a rack and let cool completely.

303 CINNAMON STARS

Prep: 10 minutes   Chill: 2 hours   Stand: 2 hours
Bake: 19 to 25 minutes   Makes: about 24

2 egg whites	2 cups ground natural
½ teaspoon cream of tartar	almonds
⅛ teaspoon salt	1 tablespoon cinnamon
1 cup sugar	½ teaspoon almond extract

1. In a small bowl, beat egg whites, cream of tartar, and salt with an electric mixer on high speed until frothy. Very slowly beat in sugar, a little at a time, until all has been incorporated and soft peaks form when beaters are raised. Set aside ¼ cup for glaze.

2. Fold ground almonds, cinnamon, and almond extract into beaten egg whites. Cover and refrigerate dough and reserved glaze 2 to 3 hours, or until very firm.

3. Between floured sheets of wax paper, roll out dough ¼ inch thick. Cut out cookies using a 2½-inch star cutter. Place 1 inch apart on lightly greased cookie sheets. Let stand at room temperature 2 hours. Brush stars with reserved glaze.

4. Preheat oven to 300°F. and bake stars 12 to 15 minutes. Remove stars from oven and brush again with reserved glaze. Return to oven and bake 7 to 10 minutes longer, or until firm. Let cookies cool 2 minutes on sheets, then remove to racks and let cool completely. Store in a tightly covered container.

304 MINCEMEAT MOUNDS

Prep: 10 minutes   Bake: 10 to 12 minutes   Makes: about 36

1 stick (4 ounces) butter,	½ teaspoon salt
softened	½ teaspoon freshly ground
½ cup sugar	black pepper
1 egg	1 teaspoon cinnamon
1 cup mincemeat	½ teaspoon grated nutmeg
1¼ cups flour	¼ teaspoon ground ginger
½ teaspoon baking soda	½ cup chopped walnuts

1. Preheat oven to 350°F. In a medium bowl, beat butter and sugar with an electric mixer on medium speed until creamy. Blend in egg. Add mincemeat and beat on low speed until mixed.

2. Mix flour, baking soda, salt, pepper, cinnamon, nutmeg, and ginger and beat into mincemeat mixture until well blended. Stir in walnuts.

3. Drop by tablespoonfuls 2 inches apart onto greased cookie sheets. Bake 10 to 12 minutes. Let cookies cool on sheets 2 minutes, then remove to a rack and let cool completely.

305 POPPY-PRUNE HAMANTASCHEN

Prep: 20 minutes   Chill: 1 hour   Cook: 30 minutes
Bake: 15 to 20 minutes   Makes: about 48

2 cups flour
¼ cup plus 2 tablespoons sugar
2 teaspoons baking powder
Pinch of salt
1½ sticks (6 ounces) butter, chilled and cut into pieces
3 tablespoons grated lemon zest
¼ cup poppy seeds

2 eggs
3 tablespoons orange juice
⅓ cup pitted prunes
½ juice orange, thinly sliced and pitted
1 tablespoon honey
1 tablespoon lemon juice
⅛ teaspoon grated nutmeg
¼ cup coarsely chopped almonds

1. In a food processor, pulse flour, sugar, baking powder, salt, butter, and lemon zest until mixture resembles coarse cornmeal.

2. Add poppy seeds, eggs, and 1 tablespoon orange juice; process just until dough forms a ball around blades. If dough is too sticky, add a bit more flour. Wrap dough in wax paper and refrigerate about 1 hour, until firm, or overnight.

3. In a small saucepan, combine prunes, orange slices, and remaining 2 tablespoons orange juice. Bring to a boil, reduce heat to low, cover, and simmer 30 minutes, or until prunes are soft and orange rind is tender. Remove from heat; let cool slightly.

4. In a blender or food processor, combine cooled prune-orange mixture with honey, lemon juice, and nutmeg. Pulse until orange rind is chopped and mixture is blended but not smooth. Stir in almonds.

5. Preheat oven to 350°F. On a lightly floured surface or between pieces of wax paper, roll out dough to ¼-inch thickness. Using a 2¼-inch round biscuit cutter or rim of a glass, cut dough into circles. Reroll and cut scraps. Place 1 teaspoon of filling in center of each circle. To form tricornered shape, fold 2 sides of circle over filling, then fold up bottom to form triangle. Firmly pinch edges together. Place about 1½ inches apart on greased cookie sheets.

6. Bake 15 to 20 minutes, until golden. Remove to a rack and let cool completely.

306 CREAM CHEESE HAMANTASCHEN

Prep: 20 minutes   Chill: 1 hour   Bake: 15 to 20 minutes
Makes: about 30

4 ounces cream cheese, softened	¼ teaspoon salt
1 stick (4 ounces) butter, softened	1 cup poppy seeds
	¼ cup raisins
1 cup flour	¼ cup honey
¼ cup sugar	1 egg
1 tablespoon grated orange zest	1½ teaspoons grated lemon zest
	¼ teaspoon cinnamon

1. In a food processor, combine cream cheese, butter, flour, 2 tablespoons sugar, orange zest, and salt. Process until dough forms a ball around blades. Wrap dough in wax paper and refrigerate about 1 hour, until firm, or overnight.

2. In a blender or food processor, combine poppy seeds, raisins, honey, remaining 2 tablespoons sugar, egg, lemon zest, and cinnamon. Pulse until raisins are chopped and filling is well mixed. Do not overprocess to a paste.

3. Preheat oven to 400°F. On a lightly floured surface or between pieces of wax paper, roll out dough to ¼ inch thickness. Using a 2¼-inch round biscuit cutter or an inverted glass, cut dough into circles. Reroll and cut scraps.

4. Place 1 teaspoon of filling in center of each circle. To form tricornered shape, fold 2 sides of circle over filling, then fold up bottom to form a triangle. Firmly pinch edges together. Place about 1½ inches apart on greased cookie sheets.

5. Bake 15 to 20 minutes, until golden. Remove to rack and let cool completely before serving.

307 ORANGE-POPPY HAMANTASCHEN

Prep: 25 minutes   Bake: 15 to 20 minutes   Makes: about 36

2 cups flour	1 teaspoon vanilla extract
1½ teaspoons baking powder	1 cup poppy seeds
¼ teaspoon salt	½ cup walnuts
½ cup plus 2 tablespoons sugar	¼ cup raisins
¼ cup vegetable oil	¼ cup honey
3 eggs	1½ teaspoons grated lemon zest
1 tablespoon grated orange zest	¼ teaspoon cinnamon

1. In a food processor, combine flour, baking powder, salt, ½ cup sugar, oil, 2 eggs, orange zest, and vanilla. Mix until well blended. Remove from processor, form into a ball, and knead a few times. Dough should not be sticky.

2. In a blender or food processor, combine poppy seeds, walnuts, raisins, honey, remaining 2 tablespoons sugar, lemon zest, cinnamon, and remaining egg. Pulse until well mixed. Do not overprocess; filling should have texture, not be smooth.

3. Preheat oven to 350°F. On a lightly floured surface or between pieces of wax paper, roll out dough to ¼-inch thickness. Using a 2¼-inch round biscuit cutter or an inverted glass, cut dough into circles. Reroll and cut scraps.

4. Place 1 teaspoon of filling in center of each circle. To form tricornered shape, fold 2 sides of circle over filling, then fold up bottom to form a triangle. Firmly pinch edges together. Place about 1½ inches apart on greased cookie sheets.

5. Bake 15 to 20 minutes, until golden. Remove to a rack and let cool completely.

---

308 KRINGLES

Prep: 10 minutes   Chill: 30 minutes   Bake: 12 to 15 minutes
Makes: about 48

The flavor of these Eastern European Christmas cookies deepens if they are stored for a few days before serving.

¾ cup granulated sugar	2 cups flour
1 stick (4 ounces) butter, softened	2 teaspoons baking powder
	¼ teaspoon salt
1 egg	2 tablespoons powdered sugar
¼ cup brandy	
1 teaspoon caraway seeds	

1. In a large bowl, beat granulated sugar and butter with an electric mixer on medium speed until well blended. Beat in egg, brandy, and caraway seeds until light and fluffy.

2. Combine flour, baking powder, and salt and beat in on low speed until dough is smooth, scraping down side of bowl frequently with a rubber spatula. Wrap and refrigerate dough 30 minutes, until firm. If chilled longer, set dough out to soften slightly before rolling.

3. Preheat oven to 350°F. Between pieces of wax paper, roll out dough ¼ inch thick. Cut out cookies with 3-inch crescent-shaped cutters. Reroll scraps to make additional cookies. Place cookies 2 inches apart on lightly greased cookie sheets. Sprinkle with powdered sugar.

4. Bake 12 to 15 minutes, or until edges are golden brown. Let cookies cool 2 minutes on sheets, then remove to racks and let cool completely. Store in a tightly covered container.

309   HOLIDAY MINT MERINGUES

Prep: 10 minutes   Bake: 50 minutes   Makes: about 42

These minty low-fat confections are a wonderful addition to any holiday table.

Vegetable cooking spray
2 egg whites
⅛ teaspoon cream of tartar
⅔ cup superfine sugar

½ teaspoon vanilla extract
½ teaspoon peppermint extract
½ cup semisweet mint chocolate chips

1. Preheat oven to 275°F. Line 2 cookie sheets with foil and coat foil with vegetable cooking spray.

2. In a medium bowl, beat egg whites and cream of tartar with an electric mixer on medium speed until soft peaks form. Turn mixer to high and gradually beat in sugar until glossy, stiff peaks form. Beat in vanilla and peppermint extract. Gently but quickly fold in chocolate chips. Drop by teaspoonfuls 1 inch apart onto prepared cookie sheets.

3. Bake 25 minutes. Reduce oven temperature to 250°F. and bake 25 minutes longer. Remove to a rack and let cool completely. Store in an airtight tin.

310   HOLIDAY LEMON DROPS

Prep: 10 minutes   Bake: 20 to 25 minutes   Makes: about 48

These holiday cookies are creamy, light, and lemony—great for an assorted cookie tray.

1½ sticks (6 ounces) butter, softened
1 (3-ounce) package cream cheese, softened
¾ cup granulated sugar
½ teaspoon vanilla extract

½ teaspoon lemon extract
2 teaspoons grated lemon zest
2 cups cake flour
¼ teaspoon salt
½ cup finely chopped walnuts
½ cup powdered sugar

1. Preheat oven to 300°F. In a medium bowl, beat butter, cream cheese, and granulated sugar with an electric mixer on medium speed until light and fluffy. Beat in vanilla, lemon extract, and lemon zest.

2. Add cake flour and salt and beat on low speed until blended. Stir in walnuts. Drop by teaspoonfuls 2 inches apart onto ungreased cookie sheets.

3. Bake 20 to 25 minutes, until set but not browned. Let cookies cool on sheets 2 minutes. Roll in powdered sugar, transfer to a rack, and let cool completely.

311 MOLASSES CRISPS

Prep: 15 minutes   Chill: 30 minutes   Bake: 6 to 8 minutes
Makes: about 60

1 stick (4 ounces) butter, softened
½ cup firmly packed dark brown sugar
1 teaspoon vanilla extract
1 teaspoon cinnamon
1 teaspoon ground ginger
½ teaspoon ground mace

¼ teaspoon ground allspice
½ cup molasses
2 cups flour
1 teaspoon baking soda
½ teaspoon baking powder
¼ teaspoon salt
1 egg, lightly beaten
¼ cup granulated sugar

1. In a medium bowl, beat butter, brown sugar, vanilla, cinnamon, ginger, mace, and allspice with an electric mixer on medium speed until light and fluffy. Gradually beat in molasses.

2. Add flour mixed with baking soda, baking powder, and salt and beat on low speed until blended. Cover dough and refrigerate 30 minutes, or overnight.

3. Preheat oven to 375°F. Between pieces of wax paper, roll out dough paper thin. Cut out cookies using a 2-inch round cutter or cut into 2-inch squares. Place 1 inch apart on greased baking sheets. Brush lightly with beaten egg and sprinkle granulated sugar on top.

4. Bake 6 to 8 minutes, or until set and golden brown. Let stand 2 minutes, then remove to a rack and let cool completely. Store in an airtight tin.

---

312 HOLIDAY THUMBPRINTS

Prep: 10 minutes   Bake: 8 to 10 minutes   Makes: about 48

2 sticks (8 ounces) butter, softened
⅔ cup sugar
1 egg

2 teaspoons vanilla extract
2 cups flour
¼ teaspoon salt
¼ cup raspberry jelly

1. Preheat oven to 375°F. In a medium bowl, beat butter and sugar with an electric mixer on medium speed until creamy. Beat in egg and vanilla until fluffy.

2. Gradually add flour and salt, beating on low speed until well blended. Shape dough into 1-inch balls. Place 2 inches apart on 2 ungreased cookie sheets. With fingertip, make an indentation in top of each cookie. Spoon about ¼ teaspoon raspberry jelly into each well.

3. Bake 8 to 10 minutes, until edges are lightly browned. Remove to a rack and let cool completely.

313 PEPPERY CHOCOLATE SNAPS

Prep: 10 minutes   Chill: 30 minutes   Bake: 10 to 12 minutes
Makes: about 48

1½ sticks (6 ounces) butter,
    softened
1¼ cups sugar
1 egg
2 teaspoons vanilla extract
1 teaspoon cinnamon
¼ teaspoon freshly ground
    black pepper

⅛ teaspoon ground cloves
4 (1-ounce) squares
    unsweetened chocolate,
    melted
1½ cups flour
1½ teaspoons baking powder
½ teaspoon salt

1. In a medium bowl, beat butter and sugar with an electric mixer on medium speed until blended. Beat in egg, vanilla, cinnamon, pepper, cloves, and melted chocolate until mixed.

2. Add flour mixed with baking powder and salt and beat on low speed until well blended. Cover and refrigerate dough until firm, about 30 minutes.

3. Preheat oven to 350°F. Shape dough into 1-inch balls and place 1 inch apart on ungreased cookie sheets. Flatten gently with bottom of a glass.

4. Bake 10 to 12 minutes, until cookies are set. Let cool on sheets 2 minutes, then remove to a rack and let cool completely.

314 PFEFFERNÜSSE

Prep: 10 minutes   Chill: 3 hours   Bake: 10 to 12 minutes
Makes: about 60

Not all pfeffernüsse contain black pepper; sometimes they are merely spicy little cookies. These get their bite from ginger.

¾ cup firmly packed brown
    sugar
1 stick (4 ounces) butter,
    softened
2 tablespoons light molasses
1 teaspoon vanilla extract
½ teaspoon anise extract
1¾ cups flour

1 teaspoon baking powder
½ teaspoon baking soda
2 teaspoons ground ginger
1 teaspoon cinnamon
¼ teaspoon ground cloves
¼ teaspoon salt
½ cup powdered sugar

1. In a large bowl, beat brown sugar, butter, molasses, vanilla, and anise extract with an electric mixer on medium speed until well blended.

2. Whisk together flour, baking powder, baking soda, ginger, cinnamon, cloves, and salt. Beat into butter mixture until a stiff, crumbly dough forms, scraping down side of bowl frequently with a rubber spatula.

3. Knead dough into a ball and divide into 4 pieces. With palms of hands, roll each piece of dough on wax paper to make a 12 × ¾-inch roll. Wrap and refrigerate for at least 3 hours or up to 3 days (or freeze for up to 6 months).

4. When ready to bake cookies, preheat oven to 350°F. Slice dough roll crosswise to make ¾-inch-thick cookies. Place cookies 1 inch apart on lightly greased cookie sheets. Bake 10 to 12 minutes, or until firm and very lightly browned.

5. Place powdered sugar in a bowl. Add cookies, a few at a time, and toss to coat. Place on a rack and let cool completely. Store in a tightly covered container. These are better after a day or two of storage.

---

315 SOUR CREAM PFEFFERNÜSSE
Prep: 10 minutes   Chill: 3 hours   Bake: 8 to 10 minutes
Makes: about 60

In the past, *pfeffernüsse* was used as a generic name for any small Eastern European spice cookie.

¾ cup granulated sugar	1 teaspoon cinnamon
4 tablespoons butter, softened	½ teaspoon grated nutmeg
½ cup sour cream	½ teaspoon freshly ground
¼ cup honey	black pepper
1 teaspoon vanilla extract	¼ teaspoon ground allspice
2 cups flour	¼ teaspoon ground cloves
½ teaspoon baking soda	¼ teaspoon salt
1 teaspoon ground ginger	1 cup powdered sugar

1. In a large bowl, beat granulated sugar, butter, sour cream, honey, and vanilla with an electric mixer on medium speed until well blended.

2. Mix together flour, baking soda, ginger, cinnamon, nutmeg, pepper, all-spice, cloves, and salt. Add to sour cream mixture and beat until a soft dough forms, scraping down side of bowl frequently with a rubber spatula.

3. Divide dough into 4 pieces. With floured palms of hands, roll each piece of dough on wax paper to make a ¾-inch-thick roll 10 inches long. Wrap and refrigerate for at least 3 hours or up to 3 days (or freeze for up to 6 months).

4. When ready to bake cookies, preheat oven to 350°F. Slice dough roll crosswise to make ¾-inch-thick cookies. Place cookies 1 inch apart on lightly greased cookie sheets. Bake 8 to 10 minutes, or until firm and very lightly browned on edges.

5. In a small bowl, stir together powdered sugar and 2 tablespoons water to make a glaze. Remove cookies to a rack; brush with glaze and let cool completely. Store in a tightly covered container. These are better after a day or two of storage.

316 ROBIN'S NESTS
Prep: 10 minutes   Bake: 10 to 12 minutes   Makes: about 36

These are great for Easter. Children love to nibble on them, and they make beautiful table decorations.

¼ cup sugar	¼ cup flour
1 egg	2 cups flaked coconut
½ teaspoon vanilla extract	Jelly beans

1. Preheat oven to 350°F. In a medium bowl, beat sugar, egg, and vanilla with an electric mixer on medium speed until well blended. Beat in flour until a smooth batter forms. Fold in coconut.

2. Drop by heaping teaspoonfuls 2 inches apart onto lightly greased cookie sheets. With a floured thumb, press an indentation into the center of the coconut to resemble a nest. Bake 10 to 12 minutes, or until edges are golden brown.

3. Remove from oven and immediately press 1 to 3 jelly beans into each nest. Let nests cool 2 minutes on sheets, then remove to racks and let cool completely. Store in a tightly covered container.

---

317 SPRINGERLE
Prep: 10 minutes   Chill: 3 hours plus overnight
Bake: 15 to 18 minutes   Makes: about 36

A special wooden rolling pin and/or several molds emboss holiday designs in these traditional cookies. If you don't have the rolling pin or molds, use a regular rolling pin and cut dough into squares. These cookies are best if allowed to ripen for several weeks before serving.

2 eggs	½ teaspoon anise extract
½ teaspoon cream of tartar	2 cups cake flour
⅛ teaspoon salt	½ teaspoon baking powder
1 cup sugar	1 tablespoon aniseed
2 teaspoons grated lemon zest	

1. In a small bowl, beat eggs, cream of tartar, and salt with an electric mixer on high speed until frothy. Very slowly beat in sugar, a little at a time, until all has been incorporated and mixture is thick and lemon colored. Fold in lemon zest and anise extract.

2. Add flour mixed with baking powder and beat on low speed until dough is smooth and stiff, scraping down side of bowl frequently with a rubber spatula. Wrap and refrigerate dough 3 hours, until very firm.

3. On a lightly floured board with a floured rolling pin, roll out dough ¼ inch thick. Press design on dough with a well-floured springerle rolling pin or press with well-floured wooden springerle molds to make designs. Cut cookies apart.

4. Grease 2 cookie sheets; sprinkle aniseed evenly over sheets. Place cookies 1 inch apart on prepared cookie sheets. With a pastry brush, brush aniseed on sheets between cookies onto sides of cookies. Cover lightly with a kitchen towel and refrigerate 12 hours, or overnight.

5. Preheat oven to 375°F. Place cookies in oven; immediately reduce oven temperature to 325°F. Bake 15 to 18 minutes, or until edges just start to color. Let cookies cool 2 minutes on sheets, then remove to racks and let cool completely. Store in a tightly covered container 2 to 3 weeks before serving.

---

318 STAINED GLASS WINDOWS
Prep: 10 minutes   Chill: 2 hours   Bake: 10 to 12 minutes
Makes: about 36

Cracked hard candies melt into the prettiest clear colored windows you have ever seen. These are best if used within a week, as candy areas tend to turn cloudy.

1 stick (4 ounces) butter, softened	⅛ teaspoon salt
½ cup sugar	3 (.90-ounce) packages assorted fruit-flavored candy rings, such as Life Savers
1 egg	
½ teaspoon vanilla extract	
1½ cups flour	

1. In a medium bowl, beat butter and sugar with an electric mixer on medium speed until well blended. Beat in egg and vanilla until light and fluffy.

2. Add flour and salt and beat on low speed until dough is smooth, scraping down side of bowl frequently with a rubber spatula. Wrap and refrigerate dough 2 to 3 hours, until firm.

3. Preheat oven to 350°F. Line 2 cookie sheets with aluminum foil, shiny side up. Between pieces of wax paper, roll out dough ¼ inch thick. Cut out as many 3-inch rounds as you can. With a 1½- to 2-inch holiday cookie cutter, cut out and remove dough from center of round. Reroll scraps to make additional cookies.

4. Place cookies 2 inches apart on foil-covered cookie sheets. Separate candies by color; place each color in a plastic sandwich bag. With hammer or meat mallet, crack candies into small pieces. Arrange cracked candies inside cut-out centers of cookies, using enough to evenly cover surface.

5. Bake 10 to 12 minutes, or until edges are golden brown. Lift cookies, still on foil, to racks and let cool completely. Peel off foil; store cookies between sheets of wax paper in a tightly covered container.

319 LEBKUCHEN

Prep: 10 minutes   Chill: 1 hour   Bake: 12 to 15 minutes
Makes: about 24

In Germany and Austria, lebkuchen hearts are prepared for holidays, sporting events, and family celebrations. A string is often baked in them, so they can be worn during the celebration and eaten afterward. Plan ahead when making lebkuchen, as they improve markedly if stored several days to mellow and soften.

½ cup firmly packed brown sugar	¼ teaspoon ground cloves
½ cup honey	¼ teaspoon ground allspice
1 egg	¼ teaspoon salt
2 cups flour	½ cup finely chopped mixed candied fruit
¼ teaspoon baking soda	½ cup finely chopped walnuts
1 teaspoon grated lemon zest	½ cup powdered sugar
1 teaspoon cinnamon	1 tablespoon lemon juice
½ teaspoon grated nutmeg	

1. In a large bowl, beat brown sugar, honey, and egg with an electric mixer on medium speed until light and fluffy.

2. Combine flour, baking soda, lemon zest, cinnamon, nutmeg, cloves, allspice, and salt and beat in on low speed until dough is smooth, scraping down side of bowl frequently with a rubber spatula. Fold in chopped fruit and walnuts. Cover and refrigerate dough 1 hour, until firm.

3. Preheat oven to 350°F. Between pieces of wax paper, roll out dough ¼ inch thick. Cut out cookies with a 2½-inch cutter. Reroll scraps to make additional cookies. If rolled dough is difficult to handle, place in freezer 15 to 20 minutes before cutting.

4. Place cookies 2 inches apart on lightly greased cookie sheets. Bake 12 to 15 minutes, or until edges are golden brown. Let cookies cool 2 minutes on sheets, then remove to racks and let cool.

5. Meanwhile, prepare a glaze by stirring together powdered sugar and lemon juice. Brush glaze over warm cookies and let stand at room temperature until glaze is dry and cookies have cooled completely. Store in a tightly covered container.

Chapter 13

Quick and Easy

Actually, with the exception of some holiday and celebration cookies, many of the recipes found in other chapters in this book are quick and easy. But in this section, we've included a collection of recipes that are especially quick and easy. These cookies are for busy evenings, when you need something sweet to serve at the end of dinner or when you've promised to bring cookies and then found no time to bake them. We offer a variety of techniques that will help out. Some of the cookies in this chapter aren't baked at all. Others start with a homemade baking mix, prepared cake mixes, cookie crumbs, or frozen pastry.

You will find that many of the recipes included in this chapter are familiar to you. The need for quick and easy recipes isn't a new one. Ever since the beginning of this century, American women, juggling a home to manage, children and husband to care for, and away-from-home work to supplement the family income, have invented quick and easy solutions to "What's for dessert?"

There is always a sense of satisfaction in having created something, even when you use a shortcut. Although prepared products can fill in occasionally, homemade shows that you cared enough to create something yourself. Sweetened condensed milk was a favorite secret ingredient in many of these traditional quick treats, and it appears in some of our quick and easy ideas. Cookies made from cookie crumbs also provide a quick way to make something homemade out of a product from the store.

If you have young cooks in your home, this chapter is a good place to look for cookies they will enjoy making. Once they experience the excitement of having created a cookie by themselves, they will want to move on to more complicated recipes and a lifetime of pleasure in the kitchen.

320 AFTER-SCHOOL COOKIES
Prep: 10 minutes   Bake: 10 to 12 minutes   Makes: about 36

These easy-to-make drop cookies are the perfect after-school snack with a cold glass of milk.

1 cup flour	1 egg
¾ cup firmly packed brown sugar	⅓ cup vegetable oil
1 teaspoon baking powder	1 teaspoon vanilla extract
1 teaspoon cinnamon	¾ cup rolled oats
¼ teaspoon salt	¼ cup chopped walnuts
	¼ cup raisins

1. Preheat oven to 350°F. In a large bowl, mix together flour, brown sugar, baking powder, cinnamon, and salt. Make a well in center. Add egg, oil, and vanilla; stir until well blended. Fold in oatmeal, walnuts, and raisins.

2. Drop by heaping teaspoonfuls 2 inches apart onto lightly greased cookie sheets. Bake 10 to 12 minutes, or until golden brown. Let cookies cool 2 minutes on sheets, then remove to racks and let cool completely. Store in a tightly covered container.

---

321 JAM SESSIONS
Prep: 10 minutes   Chill: 15 minutes   Bake: 15 minutes
Makes: about 40

½ (17¼-ounce) package frozen puff pastry	¼ cup finely chopped walnuts
¾ cup granulated sugar	3 tablespoons firmly packed dark brown sugar
⅓ cup raspberry jam	2 teaspoons cinnamon

1. Thaw puff pastry according to package directions. Sprinkle ½ cup of sugar over a flat work surface. Set puff pastry sheet on sugar and top with remaining ¼ cup sugar. Roll out dough into an 11 × 14-inch rectangle. Spread jam over pastry.

2. In a small bowl, mix together walnuts, brown sugar, and cinnamon. Sprinkle over jam. With heel of hand, gently press nuts into surface. Gently roll up from a long side, like a jelly roll. Cover with plastic wrap and refrigerate 15 minutes.

3. Preheat oven to 400°F. Line 2 cookie sheets, preferably insulated, with parchment paper or foil.

4. Using a very sharp knife, cut pastry into slices ⅜ inch thick and place slices on prepared cookie sheet. Bake 15 minutes, or until golden brown. Remove to a rack and let cool completely.

322 FIVE-LAYER BARS
Prep: 5 minutes   Bake: 20 to 25 minutes   Makes: 36

1 stick (4 ounces) butter,
  melted
2 cups graham cracker crumbs
1 cup chopped walnuts
6 ounces semisweet chocolate
  chips (1 cup)

1½ cups flaked coconut
1 (14-ounce) can sweetened
  condensed milk (*not*
  evaporated milk)

1. Preheat oven to 350°F. Pour butter into bottom of 9 × 13-inch baking pan. Sprinkle graham cracker crumbs evenly over butter. Sprinkle on nuts, followed by chocolate chips and coconut. Pour condensed milk over top.

2. Bake 20 to 25 minutes, until lightly browned. Remove to a rack and let cool completely before cutting into 36 bars.

323 NO-BAKE CHOCOLATE HAZELNUT DROPS
Prep: 20 minutes   Cook: none   Chill: 2 hours   Makes: 24

The secret ingredient in these quick cookies is the European favorite, chocolate hazelnut spread, now readily available in America.

2 cups crisp rice cereal
½ cup chopped hazelnuts

⅓ cup chocolate hazelnut
  spread, such as Nutella

1. In a large bowl, combine cereal, chopped hazelnuts, and chocolate hazelnut spread. Stir until cereal is evenly coated.

2. Drop by heaping teaspoonfuls onto wax paper–lined cookie sheets to make 24 cookies. Refrigerate 2 to 3 hours, until firm.

3. Store between layers of wax paper in an airtight container in refrigerator.

324 CHOCOLATE PORCUPINES
Prep: 5 minutes   Cook: 2 to 3 minutes   Makes: about 40

This is a quick-and-easy treat that the kids will love to help you make.

12 ounces semisweet chocolate
  chips (2 cups)
1½ cups chopped peanuts or
  walnuts

2 cups thin pretzel sticks,
  broken into 1-inch pieces
¼ cup crushed chocolate-
  covered toffee bar

1. Melt chocolate in a double boiler over simmering water or in a microwave, 2 to 3 minutes. Stir in peanuts, pretzels, and crushed candy until well blended. Remove from heat.

2. Drop teaspoonfuls of chocolate mixture onto a wax paper–lined baking sheet. Let cool to room temperature. Refrigerate until ready to serve.

325   ALMOND BOW TIES
Prep: 15 minutes   Chill: 15 minutes   Bake: 15 minutes   Makes: 44

½ (17¼-ounce) package frozen puff pastry

¾ cup sugar
7 ounces almond paste

1. Thaw pastry according to package directions. Sprinkle ¼ cup sugar over a flat work surface. Set puff pastry on sugar and sprinkle remaining ¼ cup on top. Roll out dough into a 12 × 14-inch rectangle. Cut rectangle crosswise into 4 strips 3½ inches wide; then cut each strip crosswise into 12 (1-inch) pieces.

2. Between 2 pieces of wax paper, roll out almond paste into a 9 × 12-inch rectangle. Cut rectangle crosswise into 4 strips 3 inches wide; then cut each strip crosswise into 12 (¾-inch) pieces. Place an almond paste rectangle on top of each pastry strip. Pinch together in center and twist around completely to form a bow tie with almond surface facing upward. Place on parchment- or foil-lined cookie sheets, preferably insulated. Cover with plastic wrap and refrigerate 15 minutes.

3. Preheat oven to 400°F. Bake bow ties 15 minutes, or until golden brown. Remove to a rack and let cool completely.

---

326   FUDGE DROPS
Prep: 10 minutes   Cook: 2 minutes   Makes: about 24

This quick-and-easy recipe was a 1960s favorite. It can be modified with a variety of optional add-ins, such as those suggested below.

1 cup sugar
4 tablespoons butter
¼ cup milk
3 tablespoons unsweetened cocoa powder
¼ cup chunky peanut butter
½ teaspoon vanilla extract

1 cup rolled oats
½ cup unsalted peanuts
½ cup flaked coconut, raisins, chopped dates, and/or chopped mixed candied fruit (optional)

1. In a large saucepan, combine sugar, butter, milk, and cocoa powder. Bring to a boil over medium heat, stirring often. Once fully boiling, let boil 2 minutes.

2. Remove fudge mixture from heat. Stir in peanut butter and vanilla until completely combined. Then fold in oatmeal, peanuts, and any of the optional ingredients you wish.

3. Drop by heaping teaspoonfuls onto oiled wax paper. Set aside to cool completely. When cool, remove drops from wax paper and store in a tightly covered container.

327 QUICK GINGER DROPS
Prep: 4 minutes   Bake: 12 to 15 minutes   Makes: about 32

Make these sugar-topped, molasses-mellowed drops in a wink with a gingerbread mix.

1 (14-ounce) package gingerbread mix	1 egg
	1 tablespoon sugar

1. Preheat oven to 350°F. In a large bowl, beat gingerbread mix, egg, and 3 tablespoons water with an electric mixer on medium speed until a stiff dough forms. Add 1 more tablespoon water, if necessary, to make a manageable dough.

2. Drop by slightly rounded teaspoonfuls 2 inches apart onto lightly greased cookie sheets. Sprinkle sugar over tops.

3. Bake 12 to 15 minutes, or until centers are firm. Let cookies cool 2 minutes on sheets, then remove to racks and let cool completely. Store in a tightly covered container.

328 SIX-LAYER BARS
Prep: 10 minutes   Bake: 18 to 22 minutes   Makes: 25

Sweetened condensed milk is the secret ingredient in these fun-to-assemble chewy bars.

4 tablespoons butter, softened	10 ounces peanut-butter baking chips (1⅔ cups)
1½ cups graham cracker crumbs (about 24 crackers)	½ cup unsalted roasted peanuts
6 ounces chocolate chips (1 cup)	1 (14-ounce) can sweetened condensed milk (*not* evaporated milk)
1 cup puffed wheat cereal	

1. Preheat oven to 350°F. Spread butter over bottom and ½ inch up sides of a 9 × 13-inch baking pan.

2. Pat graham cracker crumbs firmly into bottom of pan. Sprinkle chocolate chips evenly over cracker crumbs, followed by a layer each of cereal, peanut-butter chips, and peanuts. Pour condensed milk evenly over top.

3. Bake 18 to 22 minutes, or until bubbly and edges are lightly browned. Do not overbake. Remove pan to a rack, immediately loosen edges, and cut into 25 bars. With a spatula, remove bars to oiled wax paper or aluminum foil and let cool completely. Store in an airtight container or wrap well and refrigerate.

329 NO-BAKE GRANOLA BARS
Prep: 10 minutes   Cook: 2 to 3 minutes   Chill: 1 hour
Makes: 9

No need to turn on the oven for this easy-to-make treat.

½ cup semisweet chocolate
   chips
⅔ cup raspberry jam
2 cups granola

½ cup toasted slivered
   almonds
½ teaspoon almond extract

1. Grease an 8-inch square pan. In a small saucepan, cook chocolate and raspberry jam over low heat, stirring constantly, until melted and smooth, 2 to 3 minutes. Remove from heat and stir in granola, almonds, and almond extract.

2. Spread mixture evenly over bottom of prepared pan. Refrigerate until firm, about 1 hour, then cut into 9 bars.

330 ORANGE SPICE PALM COOKIES
Prep: 10 minutes   Chill: 15 minutes   Bake: 15 minutes
Makes: about 40

½ (17¼-ounce) package frozen
   puff pastry
1 cup sugar

4 tablespoons butter, softened
2 teaspoons grated orange zest
2 teaspoons cinnamon

1. Thaw pastry according to package directions. Sprinkle a work surface with ½ cup sugar and top with puff pastry. Sprinkle ¼ cup sugar over pastry. Roll out dough into an 11 × 14-inch rectangle. Spread surface with butter.

2. In a small bowl, mix together remaining ¼ cup sugar with orange zest and cinnamon. Sprinkle over butter.

3. Fold each long side of pastry into center, so sides almost meet. Fold again, to bring folded edges together. Pastry should be 4 layers thick. Cover with plastic wrap and refrigerate 15 minutes.

4. Preheat oven to 400°F. Line 2 cookie sheets, preferably insulated, with parchment paper or foil.

5. Using a very sharp knife, cut pastry ⅜ inch thick and place slices on prepared cookie sheet. Bake 15 minutes, or until golden brown. Remove to a rack and let cool completely.

331 BOURBON BALLS
Prep: 20 minutes   Cook: none   Chill: 2 hours   Makes: about 48

There are many variations of this recipe. If you can wait, they will be even better after a day of storage in the refrigerator.

2 cups vanilla cookie crumbs (see Note)
1 cup finely chopped pecans
1¼ cups powdered sugar

¼ cup bourbon
3 tablespoons apricot preserves

1. In a medium bowl, combine cookie crumbs, pecans, 1 cup powdered sugar, bourbon, and apricot preserves. Stir until well blended.

2. With hands, form into 1-inch balls. Roll balls in remaining ¼ cup powdered sugar and place between layers of wax paper in a tightly covered container. Refrigerate at least 2 to 3 hours, until chilled, before serving. Store in refrigerator for up to 3 weeks.

NOTE: *Use our Cornmeal Icebox Cookies (page 75), Rolled Sugar Cookies (page 36), or purchased vanilla wafers to make crumbs.*

---

332 CHOCOLATE RUM BALLS
Prep: 20 minutes   Cook: none   Chill: 2 hours   Makes: about 48

Years ago, cooks didn't waste a thing. This is one of many old-fashioned secrets for giving new life to stale cookies. Prohibition-era cooks substituted cider for the rum.

2 cups chocolate cookie crumbs (see Note)
1 cup finely chopped walnuts
1 cup powdered sugar

¼ cup dark rum
3 tablespoons light corn syrup
¼ cup sweetened cocoa drink mix

1. In a medium bowl, combine cookie crumbs, walnuts, powdered sugar, rum, and corn syrup. Stir until well blended.

2. With hands, form into 1-inch balls. Roll balls in cocoa mix and place between layers of wax paper in a tightly covered container. Refrigerate at least 2 to 3 hours, until chilled, before serving. Store in refrigerator for up to 3 weeks.

NOTE: *Use our Chocolate-Walnut Slices (page 73), Chocolate Wafers (page 54), or purchased chocolate wafer cookies.*

333 MARSHMALLOW CEREAL DROPS

Prep: 10 minutes   Cook: 2 minutes   Makes: about 36

Everyone loves these sticky, finger-licking cookies. They are almost as much fun to make as to eat.

½ (10-ounce) package large
    marshmallows (about 24)
2 tablespoons butter
1 teaspoon vanilla extract
1 cup cornflakes

1 cup crisp rice cereal
1 cup ring-shaped oat cereal
½ cup chopped walnuts
¼ cup raisins

1. In a large saucepan, warm marshmallows and butter over very low heat, stirring occasionally, until melted, about 2 minutes. Remove from heat and stir in vanilla.

2. Add cornflakes, rice, and oat cereals, nuts, and raisins all at once. Stir until combined.

3. Using 2 well-buttered teaspoons, drop by teaspoonfuls ½ inch apart onto generously greased cookie sheets or aluminum foil. Let cookies cool completely at room temperature. Store between layers of wax paper in a tightly covered container.

334 QUICK MOLASSES RAISIN COOKIES

Prep: 4 minutes   Bake: 12 to 15 minutes   Makes: about 18

A quick version of the old-fashioned soft molasses-raisin cookie that Grandma used to make.

1 (14-ounce) package
    gingerbread mix

1 egg
⅓ cup raisins

1. Preheat oven to 350°F. In a large bowl, beat gingerbread mix, egg, and ⅓ cup water with an electric mixer on medium speed until a soft dough forms. Fold in raisins.

2. Drop by slightly rounded measuring tablespoonfuls 2 inches apart onto lightly greased cookie sheets.

3. Bake 12 to 15 minutes, or until centers are firm. Let cookies cool 2 minutes on sheets, then remove to racks and let cool completely. Store in a tightly covered container.

335 NUTTY DISCOS

Prep: 10 minutes   Chill: 15 minutes   Bake: 15 minutes
Makes: about 40

½ (17¼-ounce) package frozen
  puff pastry
¾ cup granulated sugar
4 tablespoons butter, softened

¼ cup firmly packed dark
  brown sugar
¼ cup finely chopped walnuts
2 teaspoons cinnamon

1. Thaw puff pastry according to package directions. Sprinkle ½ cup sugar over a flat work surface. Set puff pastry on sugar and sprinkle remaining ¼ cup on top. Roll out dough into an 11 × 14-inch rectangle. Spread softened butter over pastry.

2. In a small bowl, mix together brown sugar, walnuts, and cinnamon. Sprinkle over butter. With heel of hand, gently press nuts into surface. Gently roll up from a long side, like a jelly roll. Cover with plastic wrap and refrigerate 15 minutes.

3. Preheat oven to 400°F. Line 2 cookie sheets, preferably insulated, with parchment paper or foil.

4. Using a very sharp knife, cut pastry ⅜ inch thick and place slices on prepared cookie sheet. Bake 15 minutes, or until golden brown. Remove to a rack and let cool completely.

336 AMARETTI KISSES

Prep: 7 minutes   Cook: 2 to 3 minutes   Chill: 15 minutes
Makes: about 24

6 ounces semisweet chocolate
  chips (1 cup)
3 tablespoons butter
¼ cup powdered sugar
1 tablespoon strong brewed
  coffee

1 teaspoon almond extract
1 cup crushed amaretti
  cookies
½ cup finely chopped almonds
¼ cup unsweetened cocoa
  powder

1. In a small saucepan, combine chocolate chips, butter, powdered sugar, and coffee. Cook over low heat, stirring often, until chocolate and butter melt and mixture is smooth, 2 to 3 minutes.

2. Stir in almond extract, amaretti crumbs, and almonds. Cover with wax paper and refrigerate until almost firm, about 15 minutes.

3. Shape into 1-inch balls and roll in cocoa powder. Store in refrigerator until serving time.

337 CHOCOLATE HAZELNUT BALLS
Prep: 20 minutes   Cook: none   Chill: 2 hours   Makes: 24

1½ cups vanilla cookie crumbs (see Note)	½ cup chocolate hazelnut spread, such as Nutella
½ cup finely chopped hazelnuts	2 to 3 tablespoons unsweetened cocoa powder

1. In a medium bowl, combine cookie crumbs, hazelnuts, and hazelnut spread. Stir until well blended.

2. With hands, form into 24 balls 1 inch in diameter. Roll balls in cocoa powder and place between layers of wax paper in a tightly covered container. Refrigerate at least 2 to 3 hours, until chilled, before serving. Store in refrigerator.

NOTE: *Use our Cornmeal Icebox Cookies (page 75), Rolled Sugar Cookies (page 36), or purchased vanilla wafers to make crumbs.*

338 QUICK-MIX COOKIE MIX
Prep: 10 minutes   Makes: 7 cups mix

For homemade scratch cookies in a flash, to each cup cookie mix add ¼ cup milk and ¼ teaspoon vanilla extract. Drop by heaping teaspoonfuls 2 inches apart onto a lightly greased cookie sheet and bake in a 350°F. oven 10 to 12 minutes. Each cupful makes about 10 cookies.

2 cups all-purpose flour	½ teaspoon salt
2 cups whole wheat flour	2 sticks (8 ounces) butter, cut into chunks
2 cups sugar	
4 teaspoons baking powder	

1. In a large bowl, stir together all-purpose flour and whole wheat flour, sugar, baking powder, and salt.

2. Cut butter into flour mixture with a pastry blender or 2 knives until very fine crumbs form.

3. Store cookie mix in an airtight container in refrigerator for up to 2 months until ready to use.

339 QUICK-MIX APPLE DROP COOKIES
Prep: 5 minutes   Bake: 8 to 10 minutes   Makes: about 30

2 cups Quick-Mix Cookie Mix
(page 216)
1 teaspoon cinnamon
¼ teaspoon grated nutmeg

⅓ cup apple cider
1 small apple, finely chopped
(½ cup)
1 tablespoon cinnamon sugar

1. Preheat oven to 350°F. In a large bowl, stir together cookie mix, cinnamon, and nutmeg. Beat in cider and chopped apple until a soft dough forms.

2. Drop by heaping teaspoonfuls 2 inches apart onto lightly greased cookie sheets. Sprinkle cinnamon sugar over tops.

3. Bake 8 to 10 minutes. Let stand on cookie sheets 2 minutes to cool, then remove to a rack and let cool completely.

---

340 QUICK-MIX GINGER COOKIES
Prep: 5 minutes   Bake: 8 to 10 minutes   Makes: about 32

2½ cups Quick-Mix Cookie Mix
(page 216)
1 tablespoon ground ginger

⅓ cup vegetable oil
¼ cup light molasses

1. Preheat oven to 350°F. In a large bowl, stir together cookie mix and ginger. Beat in oil and molasses until a soft dough forms.

2. Drop by heaping teaspoonfuls 2 inches apart onto lightly greased cookie sheets.

3. Bake 8 to 10 minutes. Allow to stand on cookie sheets 2 minutes to cool, then remove to rack to cool completely.

---

341 QUICK-MIX RAISIN SPICE COOKIES
Prep: 5 minutes   Bake: 8 to 10 minutes   Makes: about 30

2 cups Quick-Mix Cookie Mix
(page 216)
1 teaspoon cinnamon

¼ teaspoon grated nutmeg
⅓ cup milk
¼ cup raisins

1. Preheat oven to 350°F. In a large bowl, stir together cookie mix, cinnamon, and nutmeg. Beat in milk and raisins until a soft dough forms.

2. Drop by heaping teaspoonfuls 2 inches apart onto lightly greased cookie sheets. Bake 8 to 10 minutes. Allow to stand on cookie sheets 2 minutes to cool, then remove to a rack and let cool completely.

342   QUICK-MIX TOFFEE BARS
Prep: 5 minutes   Bake: 20 minutes   Makes: 16

1   cup Quick-Mix Cookie Mix
    (page 216)
¼   cup vegetable oil
1   teaspoon vanilla extract
½   cup butterscotch baking
    chips

½   cup semisweet chocolate
    chips
½   cup chopped pecans

1. Preheat oven to 350°F. Grease a 9-inch square pan. In a medium bowl, stir together cookie mix, oil, and vanilla; pat into pan to make a level layer.

2. Bake 15 minutes, or until top is golden brown and a toothpick inserted in center comes out clean. Remove pan from oven; leave oven on.

3. Sprinkle butterscotch chips, chocolate chips, and pecans over dough. Return to oven and bake 5 minutes, or until chips have softened. Remove to a rack. With a spatula, swirl melted chips together. Cut into 16 bars and let cool completely. Store in an airtight container.

---

343   QUICK PEANUT BUTTER COOKIES
Prep: 7 minutes   Bake: 12 to 15 minutes   Makes: about 60

A yellow cake mix gives you a head start when preparing the dough for this family favorite.

1   (18¼-ounce) package yellow
    cake mix
1¼   cups chunky peanut butter

1   egg
    Whole salted peanuts
    (optional)

1. Preheat oven to 350°F. In a large bowl, beat cake mix, peanut butter, egg, and ⅓ cup water with an electric mixer on medium speed until a stiff dough forms. Add up to 3 tablespoons more water, if necessary, to make a manageable dough.

2. Shape dough into 1¼-inch balls; place 2 inches apart on lightly greased cookie sheets. With floured tines of a fork, press ridges into center of each. If desired, press a peanut into center of each.

3. Bake 12 to 15 minutes, or until edges are golden brown. Let cookies cool 2 minutes on sheets, then remove to racks and let cool completely. Store in a tightly covered container.

344 QUICK RAISIN SUGAR COOKIES

Prep: 5 minutes   Bake: 8 to 10 minutes   Makes: about 44

With this quick-mix idea, you can bake cookies while preparing dinner and have them warm for dessert.

1 (18¼-ounce) package yellow cake mix	½ cup raisins
1 egg	Powdered sugar

1. Preheat oven to 350°F. In a large bowl, beat cake mix, egg, and ⅓ cup water with an electric mixer on medium speed until a soft dough forms. Stir in raisins.

2. Drop by heaping measuring tablespoonfuls 3 inches apart onto lightly greased cookie sheets.

3. Bake 8 to 10 minutes, or until edges are golden brown and centers seem firm. Let cookies cool 2 minutes on sheets, then remove to racks to cool completely. Store in a tightly covered container. Dust with powdered sugar before serving.

345 QUICK RUGELACH

Prep: 10 minutes   Chill: 15 minutes   Bake: 15 minutes   Makes: 30

When you don't have time to make the dough for rugelach, use puff pastry as a quick and delicious alternative.

½ (17¼-ounce) package frozen puff pastry	¼ cup strawberry jam
1 cup sugar	¼ cup chopped walnuts
	1½ teaspoons cinnamon

1. Thaw puff pastry according to package directions. Sprinkle a work surface with ½ cup sugar and top with puff pastry. Sprinkle ¼ cup sugar over pastry. Roll out into an 11 × 14-inch rectangle. Spread jam over dough. Combine remaining ¼ cup sugar, walnuts, and cinnamon. Sprinkle over jam. With heel of hand, gently press nuts into surface.

2. Using a sharp knife or a pizza wheel, cut pastry lengthwise into 3 strips, each about 3½ inches wide; cut crosswise into 5 strips, each about 3 inches long to form 15 rectangles. Cut each rectangle in half diagonally into triangles.

3. Beginning at wide end, roll each triangle toward point, forming a crescent shape. Repeat with remaining dough. Place, point sides down, 1 inch apart on 2 baking sheets, preferably insulated, lined with parchment paper or foil. Cover with plastic wrap and refrigerate 15 minutes.

4. Preheat oven to 400°F. Bake 15 minutes, or until golden brown. Remove to a wire rack and let cool completely.

346 QUICK SHORTENIN' BREAD
Prep: 10 minutes   Bake: 12 to 15 minutes   Makes: 24

Joanne's mother, Dorothy Lamb, developed this recipe to resemble the cookies she remembered a neighbor making years ago.

½ cup sugar	2 teaspoons baking powder
1 (11-ounce) package pie crust mix	½ teaspoon salt
	3 to 4 tablespoons milk
½ cup flour	1 teaspoon vanilla extract

1. Preheat oven to 350°F. Reserve 2 tablespoons sugar in a small shallow dish. In a medium bowl, combine remaining sugar with pie crust mix, flour, baking powder, and salt. Stir to mix well. With a fork, stir in 3 tablespoons milk and vanilla until mixture forms a ball of dough. Add a little more milk if necessary to make dough manageable.

2. Shape dough into 24 balls 1¼ inches in diameter. Place balls 3 inches apart on lightly greased cookie sheets. Flatten cookies with bottom of a glass dipped in reserved sugar.

3. Bake 12 to 15 minutes, or until edges are golden brown. Let cookies cool 2 minutes on sheets, then remove to racks and let cool completely. Store in a tightly covered container.

347 SUGAR 'N' SPICE SPIRALS
Prep: 10 minutes   Chill: 15 minutes   Bake: 15 minutes
Makes: about 44

½ (17¼-ounce) package frozen puff pastry	1½ teaspoons cinnamon
	½ teaspoon grated nutmeg
¾ cup granulated sugar	½ teaspoon ground ginger
¼ cup firmly packed dark brown sugar	¼ teaspoon ground allspice
	1 egg, lightly beaten

1. Thaw puff pastry according to package directions. Sprinkle a work surface with ½ cup granulated sugar, top with puff pastry, and sprinkle top with remaining ¼ cup granulated sugar. Roll out dough into an 11 × 14-inch rectangle.

2. In a small bowl, combine brown sugar, cinnamon, nutmeg, ginger, and allspice. Brush surface of pastry with beaten egg, being careful not to let any drip down sides. Sprinkle with sugar mixture. Cut into 3½ × 1-inch strips, twisting each to make a spiral. Cover with plastic wrap and refrigerate 15 minutes.

3. Preheat oven to 400°F. Line 2 cookie sheets, preferably insulated, with parchment paper or foil.

4. Place spirals on prepared cookie sheets, pressing ends of each strip down firmly to keep from untwisting. Bake 15 minutes, or until golden brown. Remove to a rack and let cool completely.

Chapter 14

Cookie Creations

This chapter includes different things to do with either the cookie doughs or baked cookies found in the rest of the book. Kids love to construct other recipes and shapes from prepared ingredients. Cookies are very versatile; the doughs can be shaped in many ways, and baked cookies may be used as an ingredient in other recipes. Bakers and cafeteria cooks have many good recipes that recycle leftover cookies as a part of another recipe. Leftover cookies are not usually a problem around our homes, but some of these ingenious recipes are so good that we make (or buy) cookies just to prepare them.

Add a bit of fantasy to your home for the holidays with our little gingerbread house. It is attached to a cardboard frame, so it is more stable than most gingerbread houses and can be prepared in four to six hours, including drying time. Once children have completed one house, they may want to make more for inexpensive presents for their friends. To add some fantasy to dessert time, prepare our cookie cups or our cookie spirals to serve with fruit or ice cream.

Whether you make the old-fashioned icebox puddings or the upscale cookie lace doilies, this chapter encourages you to look at cookies in a different light. They're not always just little rounds or squares that go into the cookie jar, but a delicious ingredient with lots of potential, just waiting for your creativity, or your child's, to turn one thing into another or into an easy dessert.

---

348 CHOCOLATE CHIP ICE CREAM SANDWICHES
Prep: 10 minutes   Freeze: 1 hour   Makes: 16

32 chocolate chip cookies, store-bought or any of the recipes on pages 86 to 98

1 quart chocolate chip ice cream, softened
6 ounces mini chocolate chips (1 cup)

1. Arrange half of cookies on a flat surface, bottom sides up. Scoop ¼ cup softened ice cream onto each cookie. Top with another cookie. Pat chips into ice cream.

2. Wrap each in plastic wrap or wax paper. Freeze at least 1 hour, or until firm. Ice cream sandwiches keep in freezer for up to 3 days.

349 JAM SANDWICHES
Prep: 10 minutes   Cook: none   Makes: 20

½ cup black currant jam
1 tablespoon crème de cassis
   or kirsch
40 Lemon Shortbread Cookies
   (page 40)

¼ cup finely chopped
   blanched almonds

1. In a small bowl, stir together jam and liqueur until well blended.

2. Spread about 1 teaspoon jam over bottoms of 20 cookies. Sprinkle about ½ teaspoon chopped almonds over jam on each cookie. Sandwich remaining cookies on top.

350 PRALINE SUGAR COOKIES
Prep: 5 minutes   Broil: 1 to 2 minutes   Makes: 18

½ cup firmly packed
   dark brown sugar
¼ cup finely chopped pecans
2 tablespoons butter, melted

1 tablespoon milk
18 Grandma Leese's Sugar
   Cookies (page 160)

1. Preheat broiler. In a small bowl, stir together brown sugar, pecans, butter, and milk. Spread 2 teaspoonfuls on each cookie. Place on an ungreased baking sheet.

2. Broil about 4 inches from heat until bubbly, 1 to 2 minutes. Remove to a rack and let cool completely before serving.

351 NUTELLA S'MORES
Prep: 5 minutes   Cook: none   Makes: 8

These are an instant treat that some very young gourmets claim is even better than the campfire version.

⅓ cup chocolate hazelnut
   spread, such as Nutella
16 graham crackers

3 tablespoons semisweet mini
   chocolate chips
½ cup marshmallow creme

1. Spread Nutella over 8 graham crackers. Sprinkle chocolate chips over Nutella.

2. Spread remaining graham crackers with marshmallow creme. Top Nutella cracker with marshmallow creme cracker to form sandwich.

Recipe reprinted courtesy of *Nutella*.

352 S'MORES

Prep: 10 minutes   Bake: 4 minutes   Makes: 8

This classic camper's snack is easy to make in the oven using homemade or purchased graham crackers.

16 Graham Crackers,
    homemade (page 155) or
    store-bought

2 small (1-ounce) bars milk
    chocolate
8 large marshmallows

1. Preheat oven to 350°F. Arrange 8 graham crackers on lightly greased cookie sheet.

2. Break each candy bar into 4 pieces. Place 1 piece on each graham cracker. Cut each marshmallow into quarters. Arrange 4 quarters on top of chocolate on each graham cracker. Top with remaining graham crackers.

3. Bake 4 minutes, or until marshmallows and chocolate are soft. Serve immediately. These are best when warm.

PEANUTTY S'MORES

Variation: Spread peanut butter (about ¼ cup in all) over bottom layer of graham crackers before arranging on cookie sheet.

353 COOKIE CUPS

Prep: 10 minutes   Bake: 5 to 7 minutes   Makes: 12

The same easy-to-make cookie dough that is used for Cat's Tongues can be shaped into these elegant cups for serving ice cream or fresh berries.

1 recipe Cat's Tongues
    (page 168)
3 pints ice cream or 4 cups
    small fresh berries, rinsed
    and drained well

Chocolate syrup and/or
    whipped cream (optional)

1. Preheat oven to 350°F. Invert twelve 6-ounce custard cups or a 12-cup muffin pan. Butter bottoms of cups.

2. Prepare dough as directed for cat's tongues through step 2. Drop by tablespoonfuls 4 inches apart onto greased cookie sheets to form 12 rounds.

3. Place cookie sheets in oven at 5-minute intervals. Bake 5 to 7 minutes, or until golden brown at edges.

4. Let cookies cool on sheets just until set enough to move, about 1 minute, then remove, one at a time, and press, top side down, over prepared cups; let cool completely. When cool, carefully remove from cups and store in a tightly covered container.

5. To serve, place cookie cup on individual dessert plate. Scoop ice cream into cups or divide berries into cup. Serve with chocolate syrup and/or whipped cream, if desired.

354 GINGERBREAD HOUSE
Prep: 30 minutes   Bake: 12 to 15 minutes
Construction: 30 to 60 minutes   Makes: 1

Here are easy instructions for a little gingerbread house that will bring joy throughout the holiday season. The cardboard frame makes it less fragile than most.

1 recipe dough for
   Gingerbread Men and
   Women (page 195)
Paper for patterns,
   cardboard, masking tape,
   aluminum foil
Meringue powder
   (purchased)

1 pound powdered sugar
Candy sticks, hard candy,
   colored sugar, dried fruit,
   nuts
Cotton batting and artificial
   trees

1. Prepare and refrigerate gingerbread dough through step 3.

2. Make patterns: From paper, draw and cut out a 7½ × 5-inch rectangle; fold it in half lengthwise to make a 7½ × 2½-inch rectangle. Label one short edge "top" and other short edge "bottom." Along 7½-inch cut edge, measure and mark a point 4 inches up from bottom. From that mark, draw and cut a diagonal line to top folded corner. Open pattern; label it "ends." Draw and cut out a 6 × 4-inch rectangle; label "sides." Draw and cut out a 6 × 5-inch rectangle; label "base." Draw and cut out a 6¾ × 4½-inch rectangle; label "roof."

3. Make frame: From cardboard, cut out 2 ends, 2 sides, and 1 base. Working from left to right, tape together an end, a side, an end, a side; stand up to make a box. Tape securely onto base.

4. Preheat oven to 350°F. On a foil-covered cookie sheet, roll out half of dough to make a 13 × 10-inch rectangle. Trace around patterns to cut out 2 side pieces and 2 roof pieces. Repeat with remaining dough to make 2 ends. From scraps, cut out doors and windows. Using knife, score gingerbread pieces to resemble wood shingles, bricks, or stone. Place doors and windows on gingerbread pieces; score to resemble doors and windows.

5. Place gingerbread in oven still side by side on foil-covered sheets. Bake 12 to 15 minutes, or until firm and golden brown. While still warm, measure against patterns and trim off excess caused by expansion during baking. Cool gingerbread on flat surface.

6. Prepare royal frosting from meringue powder and powdered sugar using recipe on meringue powder container. Spread some royal frosting on cardboard frames. Press gingerbread end and side pieces onto frames. Tie a piece of yarn, string, or ribbon around house to hold gingerbread in place until secure. Pipe some frosting along top edges of sides to attach roof. Press roof pieces into place; prop with cans or small boxes. Set aside at least 30 minutes.

7. When gingerbread is securely fastened, remove yarn. Spoon some frosting into decorating bag fitted with ¼-inch-wide round or star tip. Pipe a border at all corners of buildings, under eaves of house, and at point of roof. Decorate with frosting, candy, dried fruit, or nuts. Set aside several hours or overnight to dry. Display on cotton batting surrounded by artificial trees.

---

355 ICE CREAM CONES
Prep: 10 minutes   Bake: 12 to 15 minutes   Makes: about 15

The chocolate coating on the inside of these homemade ice cream cones makes them dripless as well as extraordinarily delicious.

1 recipe Krumkakes, page 172	6 ounces semisweet chocolate, melted

1. Prepare krumkakes according to recipe directions, but as soon as they are cooked, remove krumkakes from iron and roll into a cone with a tightly closed point. Place cones, seam side down, on a wire rack until completely cooled.

2. With a small pastry brush, brush insides of cones with chocolate, making sure that point and any open seams are coated thickly enough to seal. Let cool completely. Store in a tightly covered container.

---

356 CHOCOLATE NAPOLEONS
Prep: 10 minutes   Bake: 6 to 8 minutes   Chill: overnight   Makes: 16

1 recipe Chocolate Snaps (page 12)	3 tablespoons seedless red raspberry preserves
1 (3-ounce) package cream cheese, softened	

1. Preheat oven to 350°F. Line a cookie sheet with aluminum foil and grease foil. Prepare chocolate snaps batter through step 2.

2. Spread batter to form a 12-inch square on foil-lined cookie sheet. Bake 6 to 8 minutes, or until firm in center. Immediately cut into 4 (6-inch) squares. Let cool 1 minute on sheet, then remove chocolate squares to a rack, still on foil, and let cool completely.

3. Beat together cream cheese and raspberry preserves until blended. Peel foil from backs of chocolate squares. Divide cream-cheese mixture onto tops of 3 cookie squares; spread to cover. Stack layers, placing layer without cheese mixture on top. Wrap tightly and refrigerate overnight.

4. Next day, cut into 16 squares. Store in a tightly covered container in refrigerator.

357 APPLE GRAHAM COOKIE PUDDING
Prep: 10 minutes   Chill: 12 hours   Makes: 8 servings

This easy version of a traditional Scandinavian dessert uses homemade graham crackers.

3 cups chunky applesauce	2 tablespoons chopped
1 teaspoon cinnamon	walnuts
12 squares Graham Crackers (page 155)	

1. In a small bowl, combine applesauce and cinnamon. Stir to mix well.

2. Spread a layer of cinnamon applesauce over bottom of a 1½-quart shallow casserole; top with a layer of graham crackers. Continue layering applesauce and graham crackers until all have been used. End with a layer of applesauce. Sprinkle walnuts over top. Cover tightly and refrigerate 12 hours.

3. To serve, spoon pudding into individual serving bowls. Store any leftovers in refrigerator.

358 BANANA ICEBOX COOKIE PUDDING
Prep: 10 minutes   Chill: 12 hours   Makes: 8 servings

This is our easy version of the famous banana pudding that used to appear on vanilla wafer boxes.

1 cup heavy cream	2 bananas
2 tablespoons powdered sugar	2 teaspoons lemon juice
½ teaspoon almond extract	24 Cornmeal Icebox Cookies (page 75)

1. In a medium bowl, beat cream, powdered sugar, and almond extract with an electric mixer on medium speed until stiff peaks form. Slice 1 banana into a small bowl and toss with 1 teaspoon lemon juice.

2. Spread a layer of whipped cream over bottom of a shallow 1½-quart casserole. Arrange a single layer of cookies on cream, breaking some cookies into pieces to fill spaces. Spread cookies with some more whipped cream and top with bananas. Continue layering cookies, cream, and banana slices until all cookies have been used. End with a layer of whipped cream. Cover tightly and refrigerate 12 hours.

3. Just before serving, slice remaining banana. Toss with remaining lemon juice and arrange slices over top of pudding.

4. To serve, spoon pudding into individual serving bowls. Store any leftovers in refrigerator.

359 CHOCOLATE-FILLED LEMON SHORTBREAD COOKIES

Prep: 10 minutes   Cook: 1 minute   Chill: 1 hour   Makes: 20

The chocolate cream, or ganache, used to fill these cookies also makes a wonderful frosting.

½ cup heavy cream
1⅓ cups semisweet chocolate
        chips

40 Lemon Shortbread Cookies
        (page 40)

1. In a small saucepan, warm cream over medium-high heat until tiny bubbles form around edge of pan. Remove from heat, add chocolate chips, and stir until melted and smooth. Scrape chocolate cream into a medium bowl, cover, and refrigerate until thickened, about 1 hour.

2. Using a heavy-duty mixer, beat chocolate cream until fluffy. Spread about 1 tablespoon over each of 20 cookies. Sandwich with another cookie.

360 COOKIE SPIRALS

Prep: 10 minutes   Bake: 5 to 7 minutes   Makes: 24

Add these elegant spirals to a dish of ice cream or sorbet and guests will think you have spent hours creating a masterpiece.

1 recipe Cat's Tongues
      (page 168)

1 tablespoon powdered sugar

1. Preheat oven to 350°F. Grease handles of at least 4 wooden spoons, ⅜-inch knitting needles, or other ⅜-inch-thick cylinders. Prepare cat's tongues according to recipe.

2. Spoon dough into a pastry bag fitted with a ⅜-inch open tip and pipe onto greased cookie sheets to form four ½ × 6-inch strips 3 inches apart. Place cookie sheets in oven at 5- to 10-minute intervals so you have time to form 4 spirals before next pan is ready to come out.

3. Bake 5 to 7 minutes, or until golden brown at edges. Let cookies cool ½ minute on sheets. When just cool enough to move, carefully remove strips and twist gently around greased handles of 4 wooden spoons or thick knitting needles. Let cool until set, about 1 minute. Slide off and repeat until all cookies are formed. Sift powdered sugar over cookies and store in a tightly covered container.

361 CHOCOLATE GRAHAM DROPS
Prep: 5 minutes   Chill: 30 minutes   Cook: none   Makes: about 24

2 cups graham cracker crumbs (about 32 crackers)
1 cup plus 1 tablespoon powdered sugar
1 cup pecan pieces
6 ounces semisweet chocolate chips (1 cup)

3 tablespoons unsweetened cocoa powder
2 tablespoons butter, melted
2 tablespoons light corn syrup
2 teaspoons vanilla extract

1. In a food processor, pulse together graham cracker crumbs, 1 cup powdered sugar, pecans, chocolate chips, and 2 tablespoons cocoa powder until nuts and chips are finely ground.

2. Add butter, corn syrup, vanilla, and 1½ teaspoons water. Pulse to blend well. Form into 1-inch balls.

3. In a shallow bowl, blend remaining 1 tablespoon each cocoa powder and powdered sugar. Roll balls in cocoa sugar to coat lightly. Refrigerate 30 minutes, until firm.

362 CHOCOLATE ICEBOX COOKIE CAKE
Prep: 10 minutes   Chill: 12 hours   Cook: none   Serves: 10

Children love making and eating this easy chocolate dessert. It's the twelve-hour wait for the cookies to soften that is hard to take. To make this extra easy and quick, use store-bought chocolate wafer cookies in place of the homemade.

1 cup heavy cream
2 tablespoons powdered sugar
1 teaspoon vanilla extract

36 Chocolate Wafers (page 54)
2 tablespoons chopped walnuts

1. In a medium bowl, beat cream, powdered sugar, and vanilla with an electric mixer on medium speed until stiff peaks form.

2. Spread a thin layer of whipped cream on a serving platter to make a 10 × 4-inch rectangle. Frost 6 cookies together in a stack; repeat with remaining cookies to make 6 stacks. Place cookie stacks on their sides into cream on platter to make 2 long rolls of 18 cookies each. Frost between stacks with some whipped cream.

3. Frost entire "cake" with remaining whipped cream, pressing cream between rolls to make level top surface. Sprinkle nuts over top. Cover tightly and refrigerate 12 hours.

4. To serve, cut diagonally into slices, starting at one corner. Store any leftovers in refrigerator.

363 LACE DOILY COOKIES
Prep: 10 minutes   Bake: 6 to 8 minutes   Makes: 8

These are lovely served on dessert plates with a light dusting of powdered sugar and a scoop of ice cream or fresh berries and chocolate sauce. Or make 16 smaller doilies and place on top of 3 small scoops of ice cream or sorbet on dessert plates, then dust with powdered sugar.

1 recipe Chocolate Snaps dough (page 12)	1 tablespoon powdered sugar

1. Heat oven to 350°F. Prepare chocolate snaps dough through step 2.

2. Spoon dough into a pastry bag fitted with a ⅛-inch open tip. Pipe dough onto one half of a well-greased cookie sheet to make a free-form round about 6 inches in diameter. Inside round, pipe a spiral of circles and a web of free-form lines, being careful to touch original circle frequently so doily will stay together once baked. Repeat to make 2 doilies on each cookie sheet.

3. Bake no more than 2 cookie sheets at a time 6 to 8 minutes, or until firm and top surface looks dry. Remove from oven and immediately loosen and slide onto racks to cool completely. Repeat until all doilies have been baked. Store in a tightly covered container. Serve sprinkled with powdered sugar.

---

364 LEMON COOKIE–FROZEN YOGURT SANDWICHES
Prep: 10 minutes   Freeze: 1 hour   Makes: 12

24 Chocolate Chunk Lemon Dreams (page 91)	1 cup mini chocolate chips (6 ounces)
1 quart frozen vanilla yogurt, softened	

1. Arrange half of cookies on flat surface, bottom sides up. Scoop ⅓ cup softened yogurt onto each cookie. Top with another cookie. Pat chips around edges of yogurt.

2. Wrap each sandwich in plastic wrap or wax paper. Freeze 1 hour, or until firm. Frozen yogurt sandwiches keep well for up to 3 days.

HINTS: *When making cookies for frozen ice cream or yogurt sandwiches, roll them into similar-sized balls before baking to ensure even-sized cookies.*

365   WORLD'S EASIEST FUDGE SQUARES

Prep: 10 minutes   Chill: 2 hours   Cook: none   Makes: 24

Serve these as cookies or candy. No one will know that you didn't stand over a hot stove for hours to make them.

2 cups chocolate cookie crumbs (see Note)	¼ cup coffee-flavored liqueur
2 tablespoons instant espresso powder	1 stick (4 ounces) unsalted butter, softened
	¼ teaspoon salt

1. In a food processor, process cookie crumbs until finely ground. In a small cup, dissolve espresso powder in 2 teaspoons water. Stir in liqueur. Add coffee liquid, butter, and salt to cookie crumbs. Blend well.

2. Line an 8-inch loaf pan with aluminum foil. Pat mixture firmly into pan and level top. Chill fudge until firm, 2 to 3 hours.

3. Lift fudge from pan still on foil. Place on cutting board and cut into 24 pieces. Remove from foil and place between layers of wax paper in a tightly covered container. Store in refrigerator.

NOTE: *Use our Chocolate-Walnut Slices (page 73), Chocolate Wafers (page 54), or purchased chocolate wafer cookies.*

Index

Acknowledgments

For our children, Claire, Heather, Eric, Bryan, whose palates we've finally pleased.

A special thanks to our friends and family, who shared both their recipes and ideas, as well as their taste buds with us.

About the Authors

Joanne Lamb Hayes is food editor of *Country Living* magazine and co-author, with Bonnie Tandy Leblang, of *Rice* and *The Weekend Kitchen*. Leblang, a syndicated newspaper columnist, is also author of *Country Entertaining*.

AT LAST IN PAPERBACK!

EAT, DRINK, AND BE MERRY!

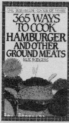

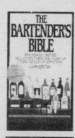

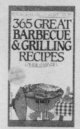

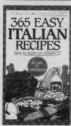

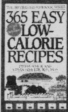

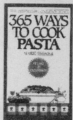

MAIL TO: **HarperCollins Publishers**
P.O. Box 588 Dunmore, PA 18512-0588
OR CALL: (800) 331-3761
Yes, please send me the books I have checked:

❑ 365 Ways to Cook Hamburger 109331-9...........$5.99 U.S./ $6.99 CAN.
❑ The Bartender's Bible 109220-7......................$5.99 U.S./ $6.99 CAN.
❑ 365 Great Barbecue & Grilling Recipes 109133-2
....$5.99 U.S./ $6.99 CAN.
❑ 365 Easy Italian Recipes 109345-9...................$5.99 U.S./ $6.99 CAN.
❑ 365 Easy Low-Calorie Recipes 109407-2.........$5.99 U.S./ $6.99 CAN.
❑ 365 Ways to Cook Pasta 109416-1...................$5.99 U.S./ $6.99 CAN.

SUBTOTAL...$_____

POSTAGE AND HANDLING.....................................$ 2.00

SALES TAX (Add applicable sales tax)....................$_____

Name_____

Address_____

City_____State_____Zip_____

Allow up to 6 weeks for delivery. (Valid in U.S. & Canada.)
Prices subject to change.   H09311

ATTENTION: ORGANIZATIONS AND CORPORATIONS

Most HarperPaperbacks are available at special quantity discounts for bulk purchases for sales promotions, premiums, or fund-raising. For information, please call or write:
Special Markets Department, HarperCollins Publishers,
10 East 53rd Street, New York, N.Y. 10022.
Telephone: (212) 207-7528. Fax: (212) 207-7222.